"*Transgender Philosophy: The Basics* is a pioneering book that is accessible, engaging, and fun. It successfully draws connections between questions of social significance that students are already interested in, and questions in metaphysics and epistemology, emphasizing why philosophy can be useful and illuminating for students and general readers alike."

Esa Díaz-León, *Associate Professor of Philosophy at the University of Barcelona, Spain*

"*Transgender Philosophy: The Basics* is the perfect book to put in the hands of anyone who wants to understand transgender philosophy, and to understand it from the viewpoint of those who actually are transgender. It's exciting, engaging, accessible, careful, gentle, and deep. Don't miss it."

Sophie Grace Chappell, *Professor of Philosophy at The Open University, UK*

TRANSGENDER PHILOSOPHY

THE BASICS

Transgender Philosophy: The Basics is an introduction to the exciting and rapidly growing world of trans philosophy.

The book covers a wide range of central themes in transgender philosophy, bringing the reader up to speed with both foundational texts and new ideas from this increasingly global tradition. It addresses key questions, including:

- What is gender? How is it related to gender identity?
- Why are we justified in believing someone when they identify as a member of a gender?
- Why do trans people transition, and how should we think about the desire to transition?
- What is the relationship between transness and colonialism, and how is it related to race?
- Should we get rid of gender? What would we look like if we didn't have genders?
- How should society be changed to improve the lives of trans people?

Accessibly written, this book offers a rigorous overview of the arguments in transgender philosophy, from abstract concerns of philosophical method to grounded and applied political issues.

Transgender Philosophy: The Basics is designed for beginners with no prior knowledge of philosophy, but it also serves a source of new insights and perspectives for students and scholars of philosophy and gender studies.

Matthew J. Cull is a postdoctoral research fellow at Trinity College Dublin, Ireland. Their work covers a variety of topics in transgender and feminist philosophy, social and political philosophy, philosophy of language, and social ontology.

The Basics

The Basics is a highly successful series of accessible guidebooks which provide an overview of the fundamental principles of a subject area in a jargon-free and undaunting format.

Intended for students approaching a subject for the first time, the books both introduce the essentials of a subject and provide an ideal springboard for further study. With over 50 titles spanning subjects from artificial intelligence (AI) to women's studies, *The Basics* are an ideal starting point for students seeking to understand a subject area.

Each text comes with recommendations for further study and gradually introduces the complexities and nuances within a subject.

PUBLIC HEALTH
Fiona Sim and Jenny Wright

SENECA
Christopher V. Trinacty

GLOBAL COMICS
Frederick Luis Aldama

CONTEMPORARY INDIA
Rekha Datta

POLYGAMY
Bruce Whitehouse and William Jankowiak

SUICIDE
Matias Gay

ROMANTICISM
Elizabeth A. Fay

LEADERSHIP
Morgen Witzel

HUMAN-COMPUTER INTERACTION
Alan Dix

ECOLOGY
Philip James

TRANSGENDER PHILOSOPHY
Matthew J. Cull

CULTURAL GEOGRAPHIES
Andrew Lapworth and Tom Roberts

For more information about this series, please visit: www.routledge.com/The-Basics/book-series/B

TRANSGENDER PHILOSOPHY

THE BASICS

Matthew J. Cull

Routledge
Taylor & Francis Group
LONDON AND NEW YORK

Designed cover image: Getty Images

First published 2027
by Routledge
4 Park Square, Milton Park, Abingdon, Oxon OX14 4RN

and by Routledge
605 Third Avenue, New York, NY 10158

Routledge is an imprint of the Taylor & Francis Group, an informa business

British Library Cataloguing-in-Publication Data
A catalogue record for this book is available from the British Library

ISBN: 978-1-032-82101-6 (hbk)
ISBN: 978-1-032-80657-0 (pbk)
ISBN: 978-1-003-50294-4 (ebk)

DOI: 10.4324/9781003502944

Typeset in Bembo
by Apex CoVantage, LLC

CONTENTS

ACKNOWLEDGEMENTS

I'd like to thank Ruth Pearce, Rach Cosker-Rowland, Filipa Melo Lopez, Federico Luzzi, Katharine Jenkins, Matilda Carpenter, Alexis Davin, Kit Heyam, and Jennifer Saul. Two groups were particularly helpful: Kevin Richardson and the students in his transgender philosophy class and the Trans and Nonbinary Philosophers Network. Thank you to everyone for their helpful suggestions, questions and feedback on the book. Thanks also to Lavender Menace Queer Books Archive for being such a warm and welcoming place to write – long may you continue to be a light in the darkness. Finally, I'd like to thank Kenneth Silver, Jade Fletcher, and Andrea Ford for many excellent and helpful conversations had whilst taking walks and drinking coffee.

INTRODUCTION

This book is an introduction to the field of transgender philosophy. Trans philosophy is a rich and swiftly developing field, with exciting developments happening all the time. More and more transgender people and their allies are stepping forward to publish fascinating works of philosophy that speak to the issues that trans people face. New insights into things like the nature of trans life, political legitimacy, the epistemology of transition, and much more are coming out seemingly every week in articles and books.

What is transgender philosophy? In the most general terms, transgender philosophy, or just trans philosophy (I'll use both terms interchangeably throughout this book), is a subfield of philosophy that brings the insights of philosophy to bear on trans people's lives and the insights of transgender life to bear on traditional philosophical issues. It asks questions about the nature of trans experience, trans people's political situation, and the cultural production of trans people. Some of the questions of trans philosophy that we'll address in this book are as follows:

- What is gender? How is it related to gender identity?
- Why are we justified in believing someone when they identify as a member of a gender?

DOI: 10.4324/9781003502944-1

- Why do trans people transition, and how should we think about the desire to transition?
- What is the relationship between transness and colonialism, and how is it related to race?
- Should we get rid of gender? What would we look like if we didn't have genders?
- How should society be changed to improve the lives of trans people?

Importantly, trans philosophy is an *emancipatory* field of study. It shares with other related areas of philosophy like feminist philosophy and antiracist philosophy a commitment to improving the lives of an oppressed group. In this case, transgender people. That's not to say that trans philosophers don't care about other oppressed groups, and indeed many are members of such groups too. One might, for instance, face oppression as a Black trans woman and begin one's philosophical work from the thought that the intersection of racism, transphobia, *and* sexism needs to be addressed. However, what makes trans philosophy distinctively *trans* philosophy is that it (at least in part) begins from a focus on trans people and their ways of life. The philosopher Talia Mae Bettcher puts it like this: "[Trans philosophy] must be undertaken, rather, with an overarching aim of exposing and combating trans oppression, of illuminating and enacting a kind of trans resistance. Otherwise, what's the point?"[1] A crucial aspect of this sort of approach to doing philosophy is that, when we do trans philosophy, we begin from trans people's perspectives, thinking about how trans people's lives might be improved. As we'll discuss in Chapter 4, this can give us a radically different way of thinking about questions when compared to those that begin from cisgender people's perspectives.

This book is an attempt to provide a 'way in' to this field – a starting point for someone looking to develop an understanding of trans philosophy – though I hope that it contains some novel insights for even the most grizzled of trans philosophy veterans. In no small part this book is a response to a demand for such a volume from people wanting to teach an undergraduate trans philosophy course but not knowing where to begin. As such, I have written this book with an undergraduate and advanced high school student in mind.

It is inspired by an introductory book on feminist philosophy that I read as an undergraduate: Jennfier Saul's *Feminism: Issues and Arguments*. That book was a vital starting point for my own development as a philosopher and continues to serve as a course book for many classes in feminist philosophy to this day. I hope that this book can fulfil a similar role for trans philosophy, inspiring a new generation of people interested in trans philosophy and keen to take its insights forward, both inside and outside of academia.

The eight chapters cover a variety of topics in trans philosophy, from metaphysics and epistemology to political theory and colonialism (don't worry if you don't know what all of those words mean yet – we'll get there). Chapter 1 looks at the nature of gender, asking what sort (or sorts!) of thing gender might be, looking at how trans philosophers have built on a longstanding feminist tradition. In particular, the chapter will focus on recent work on ontic injustice and critical gender kinds.

Chapter 2 focuses in on gender identity, something which is central to so many trans people's self-understandings, and which seems importantly different from the other aspects of gender covered in the previous chapter. Covering a variety of views, the chapter further investigates whether gender ultimately is just gender identity.

Chapter 3 turns to questions of the ethics and epistemology of self-identification. It covers debates over the nature of justifications involved in self-identification, along with questions about what we are *doing* when we ascribe or self-identify with a gender.

Chapter 4 looks at the sorts of questions that start arising when we ask, 'Why do we want to transition?' Discussing various 'explanations' of transness, before questioning whether such an explanation is desirable at all. The chapter then looks at the consequences of thinking about gender transitions as transformative experiences.

Chapter 5 is on the relationship between the histories of race and colonialism and the histories of gender and transness. Beginning by asking whether gender was a product of European colonialism, the chapter moves on to ask whether *transgender* is itself a colonial imposition on various gender-variant indigenous persons. It ends with a discussion of C. Riley Snorton's claims that gender, sex, and trans identity are bound up with the history of chattel slavery.

Chapter 6 looks at an ongoing debate in many trans circles: whether gender should be abolished. On the one hand, gender seems oppressive, but on the other, gender seems like something that is inextricable from transgender life. The chapter finishes with a look at what life might look like without gender, thinking through three radically different approaches to what we are like 'underneath' all that gender.

Chapter 7 provides a history of some of the precursors of contemporary trans philosophy, a field that sometimes goes by the name 'trans theory'. Here we'll look at figures like Susan Stryker, Sandy Stone, and Judith Butler before looking at Jay Prosser and Vivian Namaste's critiques of some of those thinkers and Paul Preciado's radical approach to gender and sexuality.

Chapter 8 concludes the book with a look at transgender political philosophy. Trans political philosophy is notable for its radicalism, and in this chapter we look at some of the reasons for this radicalism, along with two of the major strands of that radical thought: trans anarchism (as represented by Nat Raha and Mijke Van Der Drift) and trans Marxism (as represented by Leslie Feinberg). Looking at the role of history in building towards a better tomorrow, the book ends by thinking about the role of coalitions in trans liberation.

Before we get going, I also want to point readers towards the glossary. If you haven't heard of '*transfemme*' or 'if and only if' before check the glossary. There you should find a short definition to point you in the right direction. One thing to say about this glossary is that it shouldn't be taken as totally authoritative. Terminology in trans communities is changing all the time, and terminology in both philosophy and trans communities is highly contested, with huge disagreements over the precise definition of this or that term. However, the glossary will tell you how certain terms are used by many people at the time of writing (early 2026), and it should serve as a useful starting point.

Finally, a note on what I have left out and missed in this text. The eight topics surveyed in the eight chapters of this book certainly do not exhaust the rich tapestry that is trans philosophy. This is, for all its broad scope, nevertheless a partial view of the field, one that is from the point of view of a particular philosopher working in a particular tradition. I was trained in feminist and so-called 'analytic' philosophy and have lived all of my life in the Anglophone 'Global North'. Despite my continued attempts to read beyond and around those traditions, I'm sure the prejudices of my starting point show through here in this text.[2] Moreover, both the publisher and I wanted to keep this book short and readable, so necessarily many topics were left out, not least transgender aesthetics, certain areas of transgender continental philosophy (e.g., those drawing on Deleuze and phenomenology), transgender philosophy of language, and the nascent field of trans logic.

Two further topics that are perhaps especially worth noting in their absence are bioethics and the philosophy of sport. One friend was especially surprised that I left out bioethics – at the time of our discussion I was working in as a philosopher in a medical school researching transgender healthcare. However, as I continued to research transgender bioethics and transgender philosophy of sport, I kept finding that so many of the central issues of each subfield circled around one central question: Do transgender people deserve to be full members of society? In bioethics, questions about whether trans people should have access to gender-affirming care seemed to me to ultimately be about whether trans people deserve to have the healthcare that is a prerequisite for their continued existence and life in society. In the philosophy of sport, questions about trans women's participation in sports seemed to ultimately boil down to whether trans women deserve to partake in a full social life.

If there is a debate about whether trans people deserve to be full members of society, I am afraid that I want no part in it. Such questions are philosophically uninteresting, admitting of pretty straightforward answers (yes, trans people deserve to be full members of society and as such deserve to have access to healthcare which enables that and the opportunity to play sports as members of the gender they identify as). Moreover, there's also an important sense in which they are not questions *in* transgender philosophy, properly speaking. Trans philosophy begins from the assumption that trans people deserve to be full members of society, not a marginal or excluded subclass. It shares this sort of basic assumption with other areas of emancipatory philosophy like feminist and anti-racist philosophy.[3] As Bettcher puts it, "It would be bizarre to see the question whether women ought to be subjected to the rule of men as the central area of discussion in feminist philosophy".[4] Feminist philosophy begins from the assumption that women deserve to be full members of society, and anti-racist philosophy begins from the assumption that people of colour and Black people don't deserve to be treated as a marginalised class of sub-persons. So too, transgender philosophy begins from the assumption that trans people are deserving of a full and flourishing life in society.[5]

As we'll see in this book, there are plenty of debates to be had about how we should organise society and what parts of it ought to be changed or abolished. However, I begin from the moral axiom that whatever that society looks like, trans people deserve to be full members of it, free to live a fulfilling life, and treated with dignity and respect. This book is about the field of philosophy that starts from that basic moral premise and goes on to ask, "Well, where do we go from here?"

NOTES

1 Bettcher, Talia Mae. (2019). "What is Trans Philosophy?". *Hypatia* 34(4): 647.

2 C.f., Cull, Matthew J. (2026). "A Plea for Pluralism". *Transgender Studies Quarterly* and Radi, Blas, Vlaad, Sofie, Wong, Jules and Bell, Rowan. (2026). "On Trans Philosophy's Methods: A Roundtable". *Transgender Studies Quarterly.*

3 C.f., Burman, Åsa. (2023). *Nonideal Social Ontology: The Power View.* New York: Oxford University Press.

4 Bettcher, "What is Trans Philosophy?", 653.

5 That's not to say that there isn't work in these areas done by transgender people who are philosophers – I've even contributed to that literature myself defending the thought that trans men and nonbinary people deserve inclusive perinatal care (see Cull, Matthew J.; Holroyd, Jules, and Woollard, Fiona. (2025). "Caring for Everyone: Effective and Inclusive Communication in Perinatal Care". *Hypatia* 40(3): 525–546). Nor is it to say that it's impossible to do bioethics and the philosophy of sport in ways that Bettcher and I would count *as trans philosophy* (see, for example, Ashley, Florence. (2021). "Accounting for Research Fatigue in Research Ethics". *Bioethics* 35: 270–276). With that said, trans philosophy (in our sense) is remarkably uncommon in the philosophy of sport especially – at least for the moment.

1

WHAT IS *GENDER*?

Transgender philosophy, as we'll see throughout this book, concerns more than just thinking about the nature of gender. However, questions about what gets called 'the metaphysics of gender' form a central set of topics in transgender philosophy. If one of the main tasks of transgender philosophy is to make sense of issues that are at the heart of transgender lives, then it looks like making sense of gender is going to be one of the most important tasks for trans philosophy. If we want to understand what is it that we're doing when we transition genders, we probably ought to have a handle on what gender is in the first place. Is it a feature of our social lives, an aspect of our internal identities, or something else entirely? Moreover, how does this thing called 'gender' relate to sex – that is, our genitals, chromosomes, and other bodily features? Making sense of the nature of gender is a difficult task, but it seems to be something that many trans people find themselves having to come to terms with over the course of their lives. As we'll see in this chapter, transgender philosophy has put forward some powerful tools for thinking about the 'metaphysics of gender'.

'Metaphysics' is a very old field of study, going back at least to Ancient Greece. It also has a rather intimidating name. However,

DOI: 10.4324/9781003502944-2

we don't need to be too put off by this. One way to think about metaphysics is that it is a field that studies what things are, how they exist, and what their real nature is. This can be contrasted with ethics, which studies what *should* be, and epistemology, which studies *how we know* about things (more on these in later chapters). 'Things' probably sounds kind of vague, and potentially like it could cover anything: is metaphysics really that general? Well, yes! Metaphysicians study all sorts of 'things', from time and causation to tables and pregnancy. A metaphysician studying causation, for instance, might ask about the nature of cause and effect: what it is for one event to cause another? Or they might question whether causation exists at all.[1] A metaphysician studying pregnancy might ask questions about the nature of the relationship between a foetus and a pregnant organism. For example, is the foetus *contained in* the pregnant organism, or is it a *part of* that organism?[2]

In addition to thinking about the metaphysics of parts of reality like space and time, causation, and pregnancy, philosophers have also long focused on the nature of different parts of our *social* world. That is, philosophers have spent time thinking about how certain parts of our world are constructed through our shared practices in society. Philosophers like W.E.B. Dubois, for instance, have put forward views about the nature of race and whether it exists as anything other than an effect of racism.[3] Meanwhile, other philosophers have asked questions about what corporations are and whether they are the sorts of things we can hold morally responsible, in the same way that we hold most adult humans morally responsible if they do something wrong.[4]

Another aspect of our social world, *gender*, has turned into one of the central topics in social metaphysics. What is the nature of gender? Does it *really* exist? Philosophers throughout history have answered these questions in a wide variety of ways, but it is only in the 20th century that we see properly developed views about gender, largely emerging from the feminist tradition. Contemporary transgender metaphysics of gender builds on this tradition, so we'll begin there before developing the more recent work to come out of transgender philosophy.

THE SOCIAL MEANING OF SEX

Perhaps the most famous line in all of feminist philosophy is Simone de Beauvoir's claim in *The Second Sex* that "One is not born, but rather becomes, woman".[5] What does this mean? Well, one very popular interpretation is that she is claiming that sex and gender are two different things. Sex, the biological features of persons that are taken to be the basis of why we organise society into two groups (men and women), is not gender. So sure, you might be born with a vagina and ovaries, and hence have a sex, but this does not give you a gender. Having a gender, for Beauvoir, is not a biological feature of individuals but a social role that one is taught to occupy. You can be born with a penis, but you aren't born a boy: that's something that you have to learn to become.

This distinction, between sex and gender, with the former being a biological, natural phenomenon, and the latter being a feature of our social practices, has long played an important role in feminist thought. To see why, consider how the world looks if you think that gender is just sex. We live in a world where women are overwhelmingly worse off than men, face inordinate amounts of sexual violence from men, and are generally treated as second-class citizens. If being a woman is a matter of biology, then all of this patriarchal subordination is natural. Men are just naturally superior to women, and their material advantage and sexual violence is not something that we can meaningfully act to end. If patriarchy is a matter of biology, then feminist activism is doomed to failure from the start.

If, on the other hand, gender is a feature of our social practices, then there is the possibility of us acting to change those social practices. What would this sort of vision of the nature of gender look like? Well, in this view, there's biology, sex organs, and different kinds of physical bodies, *but* society makes choices to organise those bodies in different ways. Society puts people with penises in one group and people with vaginas in the other (and performs surgery on intersex children to try to ensure that they fit into one or the other group).[6] As a society, we have created and maintained practices that enable sexual violence by one group of people against another and have organised the distribution of wealth such that one group has (on average) way more than the other. Gender, according to this sort of feminist account, is this organisation of our lives, not the features of bodies that we call 'sex'. However, vitally for the feminist, things don't have to be this way! We could have a different way of organising people. We might, for instance, refuse to put people into two unequally treated groups based on whether they have a penis or not!

As such, the patriarchy can't be justified just by saying 'it's natural' or 'it's inevitable': it's not natural, and like all of our social systems, it can be changed and replaced by something different. We don't have to accept the widespread sexual violence by men against women, nor the wealth disparity between men and women, and we can fight for a society free of violence and wealth inequality. This picture, according to which gender is socially constructed and different from sex, is hence a rather attractive position for feminists!

This picture of sex and gender might be described as telling us that gender is the 'social meaning of sex'. That is, sex exists and there are different kinds of sexed bodies, but these sexed bodies only gain significance in our social lives through the practices and hierarchical organisation we call gender. There are, however, a few questions we might ask about this picture.

First, is this really the right way to think about the relationship between sex and gender? You might think that the sex/gender distinction is an important distinction to make but that we haven't quite specified the right relationship between sex and gender here. This picture tells us that there are bodies with different sexed features like penises and vaginas and that those different sexed features determine which gender the individual gets put into and how they are to be treated for their whole lives. However, this can't be quite right: it's not as if a sexist employer checks what's in someone's pants before paying them less. Instead, they'll rely on other features of the individual, like their name, their claims about their gender, their facial appearance, their dress, and so on. We need some way of making sense of this gap between sex and gendered treatment.

Second, we haven't really been told much about the nature of the social practices that make up gender. Is gender a matter of interpersonal treatment, or is it a large-scale social structure or something else entirely? We've distinguished sex from gender, but we haven't said much more about what gender actually is.

The philosopher Sally Haslanger gives us an account of gender that purports to answer both of these questions. Haslanger comes from a long tradition of materialist feminists who are primarily interested in how men as a class dominate women as a class on a large scale. For figures in this tradition like Shulamith Firestone, that men have managed to institute themselves at the top of a social hierarchy on a global scale is not something to be ignored but rather is something to be accounted for. Sure, the way that this patriarchal domination plays out might look different in different cultures, but as feminists like Firestone and Haslanger point out, this patriarchal domination is almost completely universal. Importantly, Haslanger argues, what it is to be a man is to be in this position of relative privilege when compared to women. Genders, in this sort of account, are defined as positions in a social hierarchy, and your position in that hierarchy is linked to what people (rightly or wrongly) imagine your sex to be:

> S *is a woman* [by definition, if and only if] S is systematically subordinated along some dimension (economic, political, legal, social, etc.), and S is 'marked' as a target for this treatment by observed or imagined bodily features presumed to be evidence of a female's biological role in reproduction.
>
> S *is a man* [by definition, if and only if] S is systematically privileged along some dimension (economic, political, legal, social, etc.), and S is 'marked' as a target for this treatment by observed or imagined bodily features presumed to be evidence of a male's biological role in reproduction.[7]

What's neat about these definitions of what it is to be a man and what it is to be a woman is that they give us a way of answering the two previous questions. Gender, in this account, is a large-scale social structure: an organisation of society as a whole that puts one group at the top and another at the bottom. If you fit into one of the top 'slots' you're a man, and if you find yourself on the bottom, you're a woman. Each position in the hierarchy will also come along with a variety of social roles and norms that each person in that position is supposed to fill. So, if you're in the man position in the hierarchy, you might be forced to behave in ways that prevent you from expressing many emotions, but those in the women position might be forced to do things like unpaid housework.

If you step outside of these roles or break these norms of behaviour, you'll likely face some sort of punishment (varying from the rolled eyes of your peers to interpersonal violence), and this incentivises you to keep 'in your place' in the hierarchy and in turn maintain it. This large social structure is further maintained by lots of practices of hierarchy and exclusion (from banning women from certain clubs to sexual violence), but gender is 'constituted' or made up of the structure as a whole. Meanwhile, sex does not 'directly' determine one's position in a social hierarchy. Instead, people make assumptions about what other's sexed features are: they presume and they imagine, and then they treat others on the basis of those assumptions. If such treatment is widespread and systematic, then the persons treated this way count as a member of the group in question.

Is this everything that there is to gender? Is it just a big hierarchy that applies everywhere and always, with two positions, one for men and one for women? You might think that whilst this captures something important about the way that women are oppressed in society, it is nevertheless a very coarse-grained approach to thinking about gender. That is, it doesn't quite capture the way that gender varies in local contexts and how gender operates in more complex ways than simply just the uniform oppression of women. Moreover, what are we to make of nonbinary people in this sort of account? You might think that Haslanger simply rules them out from existing from the very beginning.

Katharine Jenkins pushes a further worry: that this account of gender misgenders many trans women. To see which trans women it misgenders, let's think for a moment about three trans women: Annie, Bettie, and Carla.

> *Annie* transitioned a long time ago and most of the people in her life assume that she is a cisgender woman. People presume or imagine that she has the bodily features associated with a female biological role in reproduction and faces oppression on the basis of that assumption. Haslanger's account treats Annie

as a woman – she is oppressed and is marked for this oppression because people assume she has bodily features that are usually associated with a female role in reproduction.

Bettie, meanwhile, transitioned around the same time as Annie, but unlike Annie, makes it a prominent part of her identity that she is trans – she tells everyone. She faces a lot of oppression as an openly trans woman, but not because people think she has bodily features associated with a female biological role in reproduction. Haslanger's account won't count Bettie as a woman. After all, she isn't picked out for the oppression she faces because of people's assumptions that she has bodily features associated with a female reproductive role. Instead, she's picked out for that oppression by things like her open identification that she is a trans woman.

Carla is a closeted trans woman. She has not transitioned socially or medically and barely told anyone she knows that she would like to do so. As far as most people (wrongly) imagine, Carla is a cisgender man. As such, on Haslanger's account, Carla won't be a woman, because she isn't picked out for oppression based on people's assumptions that she has bodily features associated with a female reproductive role.

Haslanger's account thus seems to wrongly treat Bettie and Carla as not being women: it misgenders them! This seems like a serious issue for Haslanger's theory of gender. Misgendering is a moral wrong to be avoided in general, and it also has negative consequences for the sort of inclusive feminism that Haslanger wants to put forward. As Jenkins writes,

> Haslanger intends her target concept to be useful to feminists as a focal point of organizing against gender injustice. Adopting the current target concept for use in this context would therefore have the consequence of excluding and marginalizing trans women from feminist practice. Given trans women's interest in organizing against the oppression they face as women and the many important contributions trans women have made to feminism, this would be both an injustice against trans women and a severe loss to feminism itself.[8]

Perhaps, then we need to develop a more fine-grained analysis of gender than the big two-position hierarchy that Haslanger discusses.

OTHER GENDER KINDS – ÁSTA'S CONFERRALISM

One figure who draws our attention to the way that gender varies according to local contexts is the feminist philosopher Ásta. In particular, she thinks that it is important to consider how interpersonal interactions also function to give us genders:

> Consider this scenario: you work as a coder in San Francisco. You go into your office where you are one of the guys. After work you tag along with some of your friends at work to a bar. It is a very heteronormative space, and you are neither a guy nor a gal. You are an other. You walk up the street to another bar where you are a butch and expected to buy drinks for the femmes. Then you head home to your grandmother's eightieth birthday party, where you help out in the kitchen with the other women while the men smoke cigars.[9]

How should we make sense of the fact that somebody can count as a woman in one context, one of the guys in another, a butch in another context, and so on? Certainly, the picture of gender given to us by Haslanger is going to struggle to make sense of this variability in gendered treatment. According to Haslanger's account, what matters to gender is whether some person is systematically picked out for subordination based on what people think your sex is. As important as this idea is, it sets aside detailed questions about the differing treatment across contexts of that person as a butch, versus as a woman, versus as an other, versus one of the guys.

Ásta suggests that we might instead make sense of gender as a *conferred* property. That is, gender is something that is applied or given to us in various different contexts. For Ásta, when you are at work in the coding office, your coworkers confer you the gender *one of the guys.* When you are in the straight bar, you are conferred the gender *neither guy nor gal: other.* When you are in the gay bar, the staff and other patrons confer you the identity *butch.* And when you're at home with your family, they confer on you the gender *woman*. In this story, gender is about the treatment of you by others, their expectations, the standards of behaviour they impose upon you, and their perceptions of you.

How does this interpersonal conferral of gender work? Ásta suggests that people with *standing* in a context will confer on others a gender if they think that those others have the appropriate *base property*. What is standing? One way to think of it is that if you have standing, you are 'someone who matters'. If you have standing in a context, you have a degree of authority and power in that context. This authority and power (often in conjunction with others) allows you to shape the social environment. Now, in any given context, people with standing will have some idea about what they think gender is. In trans-inclusive environments, this might be something like 'what someone identifies as', meanwhile, in other contexts, people might think that what matters for determining what gender someone is is 'what sex organs someone has', perhaps 'whether one is systematically subordinated on the basis of their perceived sex', or perhaps something else. Whatever people think determines what gender you are in a given context is, in Ásta's terms, the *base property*.

In the gay bar, most of the patrons and staff will likely have standing. Not everyone, of course – the cisgender straight couple who accidentally came to the wrong bar won't have the social power to reshape what counts as gender in the bar – but those who do have standing will likely have some shared idea about what makes a someone a butch. Let's imagine that their shared base property for butchness is *self-identifies as a butch*. Those with standing will treat anyone who they think has that base property as a butch – imposing on them norms of behaviour and expectations that come along with butchness. If Ásta's story is anything to go by, this in no small part means an expectation that they will pick up the tab!

Of course, people aren't perfect judges of whether or not someone has a base property (especially when the base property in question is something like one's chromosomes or one's gender self-identification!). There are times when those with standing get it wrong and think that someone (say) has a certain arrangement of sex organs when in fact they do not. Here, they will nevertheless continue to confer that person a particular gender – at least until they come to realise that they were wrong about the person having the relevant base property. What matters, at least for Ásta, is the treatment of others as if they have that base property, not whether they actually have it.

There is much to like about Ásta's position. Unlike Haslanger's position, it can relatively easily make sense of genders beyond man and woman like nonbinary: one just has to be in a context where there are people with standing who treat you as nonbinary. Beyond this, her position is also well suited to thinking about the way that institutions impose gender upon us. Whilst in most local contexts, gender is a communal matter, conferred by those with standing in a given community, there are also plenty of situations where institutions that have the authority to confer gender. Think, for instance, of a gender marker on a passport or the gender you are assigned in a national healthcare database. In each case, some legal or healthcare institution is in charge of what gender marker goes where. These *institutional* genders operate in a similar manner to the community conferred or *communal* genders discussed previously. The institution in question will have a base property that they think matters for who counts as what gender and then confers upon people the appropriate gender, treating them as a man, woman, nonbinary, and so on.

However, you might think that there's something a little odd about gender always being something that gets imposed 'from the outside'. For Ásta, no matter whether it is institutions with authority or people with standing, gender is always something that is imposed by others upon us. You might just reject this outright, insisting that gender is something that ought to be 'up to us' in an important sense. In a view that claims that gender is just what you self-identify as, Ásta is just wrong to claim that your gender is given to you by others. Another version of this worry is that Ásta's account struggles to make sense of the 'closet'. Suppose that you identify as a woman but that you have lived for all of your life so far as a man and haven't come out to anyone: you are a closeted trans woman. As you move through the world through all sorts of different contexts, everyone treats you as a man, and all of your legal documents have an 'M' marker on them. According to Ásta's conferralism, you are a man across every context! But there is an important sense in which many of us would want to say that you are *really* a woman. Sure, you're not being treated as one right now, but you are in fact a woman. So, Ásta's account surely can't be the whole story when it comes to gender – we also need to incorporate gender as self-identification.[10] (We'll look at gender as self-identification in more detail in the next chapter.)

PLURALISM, ONTIC INJUSTICE, AND ONTOLOGICAL OPPRESSION

One response that many contemporary trans philosophers have had to this situation is to endorse gender pluralism. The thought here is a conciliatory one. Haslanger was certainly onto something when she was investigating large-scale social structures that subordinate certain groups. Meanwhile, Ásta has pointed out important ways in which interpersonal power and treatment shape our gendered lives. Moreover, there's an important sense in which gender is tied up with our self and personal identity. Perhaps all of these things are gender! There is gender as social structure, gender as interpersonal treatment, gender as self-identity, and perhaps more beyond!

Thus, if we want to answer the question 'what gender are you?' we might have different answers depending on what sense of the word 'gender' we're interested in. You might be a woman insofar as we're thinking about gender as a social structure, nonbinary insofar as we're thinking about your interpersonal treatment in your local gay bar, and agender insofar as we're asking about your self-identity. Pluralists seem, at least at first glance, to have the best of all worlds: they are able to account for all of the wide variety of things that we think of as gender. For instance, they can explain someone being in the closet as a case where someone's gender as interpersonal treatment does not match their gender self-identification because that person has not informed others about their gender self-identification.

You might think that there's something a bit troubling about this sort of position, though, because in endorsing all sorts of gender kinds, the pluralist inherits many of the problems that caused issues for accounts of those kinds. Remember Jenkins's critique of Haslanger: Haslanger's position appeared to misgender certain people, for instance, suggesting that some trans women are in fact men. Meanwhile, we could pose a similar sort of worry for Ásta's account: there are going to be some interpersonal contexts where trans women are not treated as women by those with standing and contexts where institutions with authority misgender nonbinary people. Consider, for instance, a transphobic legal system that only takes sex assigned at birth to matter for gender. In Ásta's account, trans women are not women in those interpersonal contexts, and nonbinary people are not nonbinary in the context of those institutions. So, Ásta's account looks like it misgenders people too. The pluralist will say that there is more to gender than these social structures, interpersonal contexts, and institutions, but they nevertheless think that these aspects of gender are real and important. As such, they are forced to say that yes, in terms of social structures, many trans women aren't women, and in certain interpersonal and institutional contexts, trans men are not men and nonbinary people are not nonbinary. So, it looks like the pluralist is misgendering people too!

Can the pluralist respond to this problem? One response that a number of philosophers have endorsed is to make a distinction between *descriptive* and *ameliorative* inquiry. Descriptive inquiry is an approach to making sense of the social world that aims to describe the world as it is and to describe concepts that get currently get used by people, 'warts and all'. Meanwhile, ameliorative inquiry is an approach that asks how we should organise the social world and what concepts we ought to use in making the world a better place.

How does this help the pluralist? Well, they can say that in thinking about how gender actually works in current society, we are doing descriptive inquiry. And, it turns out that actual society is a pretty bad place that misgenders trans people in many situations. As such, an adequate description of our social world is going to involve Haslanger's account of gender as a social structure precisely because it accurately reflects the misgendering of many trans women. Meanwhile, Ásta's account of interpersonal gender is a powerful way of making sense of how people with social power and institutions misgender trans people. So, the pluralist is just describing how bad things are – they're not endorsing that state of affairs! If they were doing ameliorative inquiry and suggesting that our society *ought* to feature this sort of misgendering, this criticism might stick, but they're just not doing that sort of inquiry.[11]

With this said, we might think that this sort of descriptive inquiry does give us the beginnings of a way to critique existing society. For the pluralist, existing society (often) makes it the case that trans men aren't men but are women, trans women aren't women but are men, and nonbinary people aren't nonbinary. This, they might remark, is a distinctive form of oppression, one to do with how people are socially constructed as members of categories or kinds that they shouldn't be members of, and excluded from being members of categories or kinds that they should be a part of. Recognising that such oppression occurs, and how it occurs as a part of our social lives, we can begin to criticise it and potentially even change things for the better in the future.

This sort of injustice goes by a couple of names in the trans philosophy literature – 'ontic injustice' and 'ontological oppression' – and philosophers spell it out in slightly different ways.[12] Robin Dembroff, for instance, spells (one aspect of) ontological oppression as our existing social kinds having unjust membership conditions. That is, the factors determining who gets to count as a member of a given category are wrongful in some way. They are concerned with,

> cases where the boundaries around a social kind are set up such that groups who ought to have access to kind membership (or to exit membership) do not or rarely have such access. The kind *eligible voter* provides a clear example. Historically, this kind had membership conditions that unjustly excluded anyone assigned female at birth; today, in many US states it has conditions that unjustly exclude persons with criminal records.[13]

Just as the category *eligible voter* wrongfully excluded and continues to exclude many people who ought to be members, so too Dembroff suggests, the category *man* (in many contexts) wrongly excludes many people who should be members – trans men, for instance. Moreover, it wrongly *in*cludes many trans women and nonbinary people who shouldn't be members of the category *man*.

Jenkins's account of ontic injustice emphasises slightly different things:

> **Ontic Injustice:** An individual suffers ontic injustice if and only if they are socially constructed as a member of a certain social kind where that construction consists, at least in part, of them falling under a set of social constraints and enablements that is wrongful to them.[14]

For Jenkins, when a trans woman is constructed as a man by an interpersonal context or a social structure, the trans woman has been forced into a social role (man) that enables them to do certain things and constrains them from doing others. In one sense, this is quite normal: different social roles come with different constraints and enablements. Someone who is a Catholic priest, for instance, is enabled to do certain things, like performing funerals and baptisms, but is constrained from doing other things – they must take a vow of celibacy, for example. Now, these constraints and enablements don't seem wrongful to the priest himself, who will have taken his vows willingly and endorsed them as a part of his religious practice. However, it is not going to be the case that every social role is taken on voluntarily.

Take, for instance, a trans woman who is in a transphobic work context, where those with social standing (mostly her bosses) treat her as a man. This will be wrongful for a couple of reasons, according to Jenkins. On the one hand, the particular constraints and enablements imposed upon her as a member of the category man may harm her directly: perhaps her bosses force her to wear a masculine suit as a part of her uniform, something that contributes to her gender dysphoria and causes her huge psychological distress. On the other, these constraints and enablements are also a form of *moral injury* – that is, they appear to diminish the value of a person.

What does Jenkins mean by 'moral injury'? Well, it begins from the thought that persons have a moral value in and of themselves. People *matter.* When we treat other people as if they don't matter, we create the appearance that others don't have moral value. Let's take an example: suppose that, thinking that it would be funny to do so, an acquaintance pours their scalding hot coffee over me. They don't care that I get hurt; they just wanted to laugh at my expense. I'm left shocked and burned, and immediately head to the hospital. I suffer plenty of harms or injuries as a result of their attack: I suffer the physical injury of the burns, and the psychological injury of the shock and panic that came from being attacked. Perhaps I now find it hard to trust anyone as a result of the surprise assault! However, in addition to these physical and psychological injuries, I also suffer a moral injury: in attacking me, my assailant deliberately treated me as if I don't matter. They saw me and treated me as if I had no moral worth. Instead, I was used as an object of ridicule and humiliation – I suffered a moral injury.

Of course, 'being treated as if you have less moral value' can take many forms beyond physical assault. One of these forms is being treated as a member of a group that is treated as having less moral value. For instance, if patriarchy is a systematic way of organising society that means that women are treated as having less value than men, you might think that anyone who is a woman under a patriarchy suffers a moral injury!

However, in what sense does a trans woman who is being misgendered suffer a moral injury? When she is being misgendered, she is treated as a man and subject to the constraints and enablements that come with being a member of the category *man*. Given that we live in a patriarchy that doesn't devalue the moral worth of men, surely she isn't suffering a moral injury. If anything, she's escaping moral injury by not being treated as a woman.

How might Jenkins respond to this issue? Well, one option is to say that gender harms us all. All of the constraints and enablements that come with various genders are wrongful to us, and hence we all suffer a moral injury from gender – not just women! Think, for instance, of the gendered social norms against expressing emotions (other than anger) that many men face. You might think that in addition to being psychologically harmful, this constraint diminishes the moral value of men by treating them as if important aspects of themselves don't matter and are worthy of shame. This claim, that gender is a moral injury to *everyone*, will likely appeal to some of the gender abolitionists we'll encounter in a later chapter.

However, there's something that this move seems to miss out. There seemed to be something specifically wrong with being *mis*gendered that we wanted to capture. Sure, you might think that we're all facing moral injury from gender, but isn't there something additionally going wrong when someone is misgendered? Presumably we still need some sort of story to make good sense of the wrong a trans woman being treated as a man.

One route Jenkins might take would be to argue that when they come out as women, trans women are sincerely saying something like "I am a woman, and I wish to be treated as a woman". This sincere assertion about who they are is an important thing to take seriously. To then place them under a set of constraints and enablements that go along with manhood rather than womanhood is therefore to fail to take them seriously as a moral agent with authority over their own life – it is to attack their personhood and cause them a moral injury. Recall the quite restrictive constraints faced by the Catholic priest that we discussed previously: these constraints don't constitute a moral injury to the priest precisely because he has endorsed them and chosen to live his life in accordance with them. The same can certainly not be said for a trans woman and the constraints and enablements that come with being a man!

DEMBROFF ON CRITICAL GENDER KINDS

Philosophers of gender have overwhelmingly tended to focus on the binary genders *man* and *woman*. Even when trans people are considered, the metaphysics of gender has largely focused on trans men and trans women. What about non-binary genders? We saw that one account of non-binary genders like *genderqueer* was offered by Ásta, who argued that we could see *genderqueer* as an interpersonal gender kind, conferred in appropriately inclusive contexts by communities and (very occasionally) trans-friendly institutions. However, how do non-binary people relate to the sorts of social structure that Haslanger pointed out?

One way of approaching this question that Dembroff suggests is to argue that non-binary genders like *genderqueer* and *agender* are 'critical gender kinds'. What is a critical gender kind? Dembroff gives us a neat definition:

> **Critical Gender Kinds**: For a given kind X, X is a critical gender kind relative to a given society [if and only if] X's members collectively destabilize one or more core elements of the dominant gender ideology in that society.[15]

What is meant by a 'dominant gender ideology' here? Well, the nature of 'ideology' is perhaps one of the most contested issues in philosophy (right up there with the nature of gender!). However, for our purposes here, we can think of a dominant ideology as a set of related beliefs that are taken for granted by most of society and the social practices that emerge from those beliefs. Dembroff thinks that (especially in places like the United States and Europe) one such dominant ideology is present when it comes to gender. They characterise this ideology as a way of thinking about and organising gender that has four central features:

The binary axis: The genders men and women are binary, discrete, immutable, exclusive, and exhaustive.

The biological axis: Every person essentially has a biological sex that, by virtue of nature, grounds (metaphysically explains/defines) their gender. By their natures, men have a male biological sex and women have a female biological sex.

The teleological axis: Someone's gender, by virtue of nature, determines a range of social, psychological, and physical features – e.g., sexual desire, occupation, family role, attire, comportment, personality features – that they either must (are determined to) or ought to have. Males naturally must or ought to have masculine features, females naturally must or ought to have feminine features.

The hierarchical axis: The biological and teleological features that are natural for men (as men) are incompatible with and more valuable than the features that are natural for women (as women), and naturalness is more valuable than unnaturalness.[16]

Each of these axes has come under criticism from feminists and trans people over the years (as we saw in our discussion of Haslanger and Beauvoir previously), and you might think that this gender ideology is less dominant than it once was. However, I suspect that Dembroff is right that these background assumptions are still hugely influential and troubling features of societies like the United Kingdom.

Of course, there are forms of life and a variety of genders that don't fit with this dominant gender ideology. You might think, for instance that the existence of trans men is at odds with the biological axis. The biological axis involves the belief that a person's sex naturally determines their gender, and yet trans men defy this belief, demonstrating that their supposedly natural sex does not determine their gender. Trans men's existence, then, seems like a rebuke to the dominant gender ideology. The gender kind *trans man* thus destabilises that ideology by showing that one of its central axes is not true.

Dembroff thinks that we can say a similar thing about genderqueer people. Genderqueer people's existence seems to threaten a number of the previous axes, but most distinctively, they seem to undermine the binary axis. Because they feel or desire a particular form of gender embodiment, role, or categorisation, genderqueer people do things like using gender-neutral pronouns, asserting that that they are neither men nor women, eschewing binary sexualities, employing gender non-conforming aesthetics, and much more.[17] These practices destabilise the binary axis of the dominant gender ideology described previously. Crucially, not every single genderqueer person needs to do these things – Dembroff leaves it open that one can be genderqueer without having to engage in these practices of destabilisation. Instead Dembroff thinks that it is *as a collective* that genderqueer people collectively demonstrate that any claim that these are the only two genders cannot hold. So, *genderqueer* is, according to Dembroff, a critical gender kind.

This way of thinking about *genderqueer* gives us a nice way of thinking about the relationship between ongoing resistance to a hierarchical gender binary and certain non-binary identities. These identities are the rebels collectively attempting to undermine the binary social structure and its oppressive hierarchy. However, puzzles remain, not least about the grounds, or basis of, membership in critical gender kinds. To see what I mean, think of when Ásta gave us an account of interpersonal gender kinds. Membership in these gender kinds was determined by interpersonal treatment by those with social standing or institutional authority. If those with social standing in a context treat you as a woman, then you are a woman, at least in the interpersonal kind sense. But what is the basis of membership in critical gender kinds? What determines whether or not someone is genderqueer? It cannot be, for instance, that a person is genderqueer on the basis that they employ the sorts of practice described previously which destabilise the binary axis. After all, Dembroff wants to leave open the possibility that there are genderqueer people who don't do things like developing a gender–non-conforming aesthetic. It seems like more work is needed for us to go from an account of *genderqueer* as a critical gender kind to an account of who is and who is not a member of that kind.

NOTES

1 The most famous sceptic about causation was the Scottish Enlightenment philosopher David Hume. See Hume, David. (1739/1896). *A Treatise of Human Nature*. Oxford: Clarendon Press.

2 See, for instance, Kingma, Elselijn. (2019). "Were You a Part of Your Mother?". *Mind* 128(511): 609–646.

3 Du Bois, W.E.B. (1897/1970). "The Conservation of Races", in Philip S. Foner (ed.) *W. E. B. Du Bois Speaks: Speeches and Addresses, 1890–1919*. New York: Pathfinder Press.

4 E.g., Silver, Kenneth. (2018). "Do I Think Corporations Should be Able to Vote Now?". *Journal of Business Ethics Review* 6(4): 18–23.

5 Beauvoir, Simone de. (1949/2011). *The Second Sex*, Constance Borde and Sheila Malovany-Chevallier (trans.). London: Vintage Books, p. 293.

6 See Gleeson, Juliana. (2025). *Hermaphrodite Logic: A History of Intersex Liberation*. London and New York: Verso.

7 Haslanger, Sally. (2000). "Gender and Race: (What) are They? (What) Do We Want Them to Be?". *Noûs* 34(1): 39.

8 Jenkins, Katharine. (2016). "Amelioration and Inclusion: Gender Identity and the Concept of Woman". *Ethics* 126(2): 403–404.

9 Ásta. (2018). *Categories We Live By: The Construction of Race, Gender, and Other Social Categories*. Oxford: Oxford University Press.

10 This objection is explored further in Cull, Matthew J. (2024a). "Queer Identities in Political Contexts", in Julie A. Gedro and Tonette S. Rocco (eds.) *The Routledge Companion to LGBTQ Identity in Global, Social, Political, and Work Contexts*. Abingdon: Routledge, pp. 365–376.

11 Cull, Matthew J. (2024c). *What Gender Should Be*. London: Bloomsbury, p. 108.

12 Jenkins, Katharine. (2023). *Ontology and Oppression: Race, Gender, and Social Reality*. Oxford: Oxford University Press; Dembroff, Robin. (2018). "Real Talk on the Metaphysics of Gender". *Philosophical Topics* 46(2): 21–50.

13 Dembroff, "Real Talk", 26.

14 Jenkins, *Ontology and Oppression*, 24.
15 Dembroff, Robin. (2020). "Beyond Binary: Genderqueer as Critical Gender Kind". *Philosopher's Imprint* 20(9): 12.
16 Dembroff, "Beyond Binary", 15–16.
17 Dembroff, "Beyond Binary", 13.

RECOMMENDATIONS FOR FURTHER READING

In addition to the works already cited in this chapter, some works that have been important philosophical contributions to the metaphysics of gender include:

Those looking for an excellent introduction to early debates in feminist thought about the nature of gender should turn to Allison Jaggar's classic text, *Feminist Politics and Human Nature*:

Jaggar, Alison. (1983). *Feminist Politics and Human Nature*. Sussex: Harvester Press.

The materialist feminism that inspired Haslanger's work has a long and fruitful history, with some of the most exciting texts in all of philosophy:

Firestone, Shulamith. (1970). *The Dialectic of Sex: The Case for Feminist Revolution*. New York: William Morrow.

Mackinnon, Catharine A. (1989). *Toward a Feminist Theory of the State*. Cambridge, MA: Harvard University Press.

Whilst we haven't looked much at sex in this chapter, it's worth noting that it is almost as deeply contested as gender. As we'll see later in the book, some thinkers like Judith Butler argue that sex (like gender) is socially constructed. More recently, Suzy Killmister has argued that we might need two concepts of sex: one to capture the natural features of bodies and another to make sense of sex as a social construction and feature of (especially medical) practices:

Killmister, Suzi. (2025). "What's Wrong with Gender-Critical Feminism?" *Hypatia*, first look: 1–22.

Another tradition in the metaphysics of gender that has appealed to many trans and feminist philosophers is a Wittgensteinian 'family resemblance' or 'cluster concept' approach to gender. Such an approach tries to account for the variety within gender categories whilst also holding onto the idea that there is something that unifies different genders.

Corvino, John. (2000). "Analyzing Gender". *Southwest Philosophy Review* 17(1): 173–180.

Hale, C. Jacob. (1996). "Are Lesbians Women?" *Hypatia* 11(2): 94–120.

Heyes, Cressida. (2000). *Line Drawings: Defining Woman Through Feminist Practice.* Ithaca and New York: Cornell University Press.

There have been some interesting debates about pluralism and its closely related cousin, contextualism. Some of the best papers include:

Bettcher, Talia Mae. (2013). "Trans Women and the Meaning of 'Woman'", in A. Soble, N. Power and R. Halwani (eds.) *Philosophy of Sex: Contemporary Readings*, 6th edn. Plymouth: Rowan and Littlefield, pp. 233–250.

Díaz-León, Esa. (2016). "Woman as a Politically Significant Term: A Solution to the Puzzle". *Hypatia* 31(2): 245–258.

Kevin Richardson has recently put forward an interesting extension of Jenkins and Dembroff, arguing that we can treat people being 'made impossible' as a form of ontic injustice:

Richardson, Kevin. (2022). "Exclusion and Erasure: Two Types of Ontological Oppression". *Ergo* 9(23): 603–622.

2

GENDER IDENTITY

In the last chapter, we examined gender as a social phenomenon: the roles, stereotypes, interpersonal treatment, expectations, and more that come together to give us the 'social meaning of sex'. However, when people talk about gender today, often they mean something different: gender identity. In this chapter we'll think about what gender identity is, and what relationship it has to gender as social phenomenon.

Gender identity is widely considered a vital part of the transgender experience. You may have come across references to gender identity in a number of places. People often say things like "she identifies as a woman", or "trans men have male gender identities". Meanwhile, the notion of gender identity has a role in medical contexts, with organisations like the UK's National Health Service defining gender identity as "a way to describe a person's innate sense of their own gender".[1] Gender identity even forms a part of perhaps the most widely accepted definition of what it is to be transgender: that one has a gender identity that does not match the gender that one was assigned at birth. In contrast to the social features of gender we looked at in the last chapter, gender identity is generally understood as something *internal* – it's something innate

DOI: 10.4324/9781003502944-3

or down to us as individuals, rather than something that is a feature of social systems. But what *is* this thing people call gender identity?

GENDER IDENTITY ESSENTIALISM

Sometimes, when a trans man comes out as transgender and starts living openly as a man, we might find him saying something like "I'm finally free to live as my authentic, true self". One reading of what he is saying here is something like this: at the heart of my very being, my essence, is a self which is gendered. Sure, he may have been raised as a girl, and for a long time appeared to be a woman from the outside, but he has always been a boy/man on the inside. Let's think of this as an *essentialist* account of gender identity. In this kind of account, gender identities are aspects of our essence: who we really are. This essence is something permanent. It doesn't change, whatever our outside appearance.

Essentialist accounts of gender identity give us a neat explanation of gender dysphoria. Gender dysphoria is the discomfort and psychological harms felt by those people who feel that their body and/or social life does not match their gender identity. The essentialist will say something like this: the trans person's true self does not match their body and the way they move through the social world. This mismatch means that the trans person is forced to live inauthentically, and this causes psychological discomfort, just as any inauthentic living does.

To get a handle on inauthenticity, let's take an example. Suppose that you're committed to being a punk: you despise authority, hate restrictive dress-codes, and are proud to tell 'the Man' to get stuffed at every opportunity. However, the only job you've been able to get recently has been working as a butler. At work, you're made to dress extremely formally, cover your tattoos, take out your piercings, and follow whatever orders your boss gives you. Worst of all, you are forced to pretend that you enjoy your work whilst you're doing it! This is not going to be a happy time for you: your work is making you live inauthentically. It's going to be extremely uncomfortable as best, and perhaps torturous as worst to act as if you are a formal butler when really you are a punk.

The essentialist about gender identity says that something similar is going on in the case of transgender people. In cases where trans people are forced to stay in the closet or are prevented from accessing gender-affirming treatment, trans people are forced to suppress their authentic selves. Moreover, the kind of suppression at issue is much more thorough than that faced by the punk working as a butler: it's not just during the eight-hour workday! After all, if you're trans and you feel that your body does not express who you really are, then it's 24/7 that you're stuck with a body that doesn't match your authentic self.

There are, however, a couple of problems with essentialist accounts of gender identity. The first concerns the question of whether gender identities are permanent. The essentialist account seems to be committed to the claim that our true selves are gendered, and that this is a permanent feature of our essences. So, whether one's gender identity is man, woman, nonbinary, bigender, agender, or something else, that is one's gender identity *always and forever.* Now, this does make sense of some trans people's narratives about themselves. Some trans people say that they were always the gender that they later claimed to be – that they were always a woman trapped in a man's body, for instance. Let's call this group of people 'fixies'. However, it's far from clear that every trans person sees their life in fixie terms. Some trans women, for instance, will claim that they used to be men and then became women. Let's call this group of people, who claim that their gender identity is not fixed permanently, 'shifters'.

Do the experiences of shifters pose a serious challenge for essentialists about gender identity? Well, insofar as we care about our account of gender identity mapping onto the claims of trans people about their gender identities, it looks as if the essentialist theory does poorly. However, it is open for the essentialist to say that shifters are just *wrong* about their gender identities. For example, nonbinary people who claim to have had male gender identities growing up, but who happily now identify as nonbinary are simply wrong about having had male gender identities in their childhood.

But why should we think that shifters are wrong about their gender identities? What evidence could we point to in order to show whether the essentialist is right here? It's deeply unclear how we should adjudicate this conflict, in large part because of the nature of the topic at hand. That is, we're dealing with what the essentialist has talked about as a 'true self', or an 'authentic being', or an 'essence'. These seem like remarkably mysterious things. You can't go outside and study authentic selves or essences like you can trees and trains. One can be forgiven for responding to the essentialist by saying something like "by analysing gender identity in terms of essences, you've not cleared anything up – if anything you've just introduced a more mysterious thing!" Without clarity on what these authentic selves are, one has hardly given us a satisfactory account of gender identity.

The essentialist position on gender identity, then, is mysterious, and makes tendentious claims about all gender identities being fixed. Because of this, if we want to have a rigorous account of gender identity, then we should perhaps look elsewhere.

GENDER PHENOMENOLOGY

One place that we might start is by thinking about the phenomenology of gender. 'Phenomenology' is a pretty scary word, but in this context at least, the idea is pretty simple: it's what it is like to experience something. So, the phenomenology of pain is what it feels like to be in pain, whilst the phenomenology of love is what it is like to experience being in love. One of the 20th century's most famous papers on the philosophy of mind was about the phenomenology of bats![2]

Let's think about an example to make things a little clearer. If you burn your finger, we can describe all sorts of things about that burn, from the way the skin on your finger is damaged, to the nerves in that finger sending an electrical signal to your brain, and particular nerve fibres in the brain then firing or 'lighting up'. These are all important parts of what is going on when you burn yourself, but they also miss out something important. They miss out on *what it is like for you* to be burned: The sharp feeling, followed by the ongoing painful ache, thoughts like "how could I have been so stupid as to grab that pan without an oven glove", emotions like regret and embarrassment, and other aspects of the *experience* of a burn. This 'what it is like' is the phenomenology of a burn.

One of the many interesting aspects of transgender people's narratives about their genders is that they often feature extensive discussion of the phenomenology of gender: what it is like to be a transgender woman, what it feels like to experience gender dysphoria, how someone experiences being misgendered, and so on. This gender phenomenology is often richly described and varies wildly. Even people who say that they have the same gender might have very different experiences of what it is like to be a member of that gender.

A feature of many (though certainly not all) transgender people's gender phenomenology is the feeling of being 'trapped in the wrong body'. This experience is generally described as a feeling that the body one currently has is somehow deeply wrong, and that one feels the need to escape it somehow. The philosopher Sophie Grace Chappell talks about this in terms of claustrophobia:

> For the pain and confusion that I did feel as a transgender child, a fairly suitable name – if we didn't like 'gender dysphoria' or 'dysmorphia' – would be 'the claustrophobia of the body'. You look at your body in the mirror and you think something very like: *Tear it all down and start again.*[3]

These 'born in the wrong body' narratives were influential in the beginnings of medical engagements with trans people. Indeed, the one-time preeminent medical volume on trans people, Harry Benjamin's *Transsexual Phenomenon*, featured such language as when defining the diagnostic criteria for someone to count as a "fully developed" transsexual, or a "true and full-fledged" transsexual.[4] Benjamin's case studies seem to back up this emphasis, with one named 'Ava' writing that she "just could not bear to return to the hated and dreaded male role that had me imprisoned and trapped in a body that I loathed" and another named Clara saying that she "was a woman, but was deformed by being trapped in the body of a man".[5]

As such, this sort of narrative became what medical professionals 'expected' to hear if the person in front of them was trans. If trans people didn't tell this sort of story, they risked not being seen as trans and hence in need of transition-related medical care. This led to a situation where trans people began shaping their what they said to medical professionals to match their expectations better, so that they might access the gender-affirming care they wanted.[6] There are even stories of trans people sharing Benjamin's book around in order to crib from his notes!

Does this mean that trans people don't *actually* think they're trapped in the wrong body? Is it all just a narrative tactically deployed to access gender affirming care? Well yes and no. There definitely are plenty of trans people who do experience the gender phenomenology of claustrophobia – like Clara, Ava, Chappell, and Jay Prosser, who writes, "My contention is that transsexuals continue to deploy the image of wrong embodiment because being trapped in the wrong body is just what transsexuality feels like".[7] However, not every trans person does experience feeling trapped in the wrong body. There is plenty of variety in the gender phenomenology that other trans people describe.

What do these other experiences of what it feels like to be trans look like? Some people explicitly deny a feeling of being trapped, but at the same time affirm that they want to change some aspect of their body. For instance, Harry Nicholas writes,

> I've never really resonated with the 'born in the wrong body' thing. There are times (and these times are frequent) when I have burned for a tall body, longed for a straight torso rather than an hourglass figure and dreamt of a flat rather than a busty chest. There was a time quite recently where I cried into my McDonald's Big Flavour Wrap all the way home because I felt that a penis was missing from my body . . . and my hips fell outside of most men's jeans. I found it distressing. That is my dysphoria and my reality. However, despite pain and longing some of the time, I've never really felt like my body is 'wrong'. My body is mine and it is all that I have ever known. There are things I wish I could add to it or take away, but at the same time I cannot help but feel that I was not born in the wrong body but rather in the wrong world.[8]

So, for Nicholas, his body isn't something that he's trapped in – he feels at home in the only body he's ever had. Rather, his body is just something that he'd like to make some modifications to. Yet another variation on what being trans feels like comes from

Andrea Long Chu: "Wanting to be a woman was something that descended upon me, like a tongue of fire, or an infection".[9] So, for Chu, what it is like to be a trans woman is to experience a great desire or longing.

Another example of this sort of non-'trapped in the wrong body' narrative comes from the journalist Meredith Talusan who writes that "I didn't feel particularly alienated with my body until I started presenting as female, and even then, it was more about how other people perceived me rather than some deep-seated sense that my body felt wrong".[10] So, for Talusan, there was never a question of her being trapped in the wrong body: it was a society whose perceptions made her uncomfortable.

For my own part, I often characterise my gender phenomenology as featuring an absence. That is, where others seem to experience gendered life as featuring a rich tapestry of experiences, some of which affirm one's gender, and others of which cause feelings of (say) claustrophobia, my own gender phenomenology is a feeling of alienation from gender. This alienation or lack leads me to think of myself as agender – lacking a gender.

So far, so good: everyone seems to agree that gender phenomenology exists and that it's really varied, beyond just a 'trapped in the wrong body' narrative. However, can it help us make sense of gender identity? Well, one suggestion I've discussed in the past is that gender identity just *is* gender phenomenology.[11] Having a male gender identity in this account means that you have male gender phenomenology. Meanwhile, having a genderqueer gender identity just means that you have genderqueer gender phenomenology.

Why think this kind of view is promising? Well, if we were looking for something internal to us, and moreover, something that seemed to track how people talked about their gender identifications, then it looks like saying that gender phenomenology is gender identity gets us a neat account. Another advantage is that it looks like we're able to account for the variety of narratives about people's gender identities. Why? Because gender phenomenology seems to be an important part of those narratives in the first place.

This kind of account also doesn't run into the problems faced by the essentialist account of gender identity. Phenomenology might be a little weird (you can't measure it directly with a thermometer or a tape measure after all) but gender phenomenology is no more mysterious that the phenomenology of pain or the experience of what it is like to eat chocolate. Moreover, it also fits with the narratives told by both fixies and shifters. The narratives told by fixies (those who say that their gender identity has remained fixed throughout their life) often feature them saying things like "I always felt like a boy, even as a child when I was being told that I was a girl by everyone around me". At other times their narratives often include references to odd feelings that had to be hidden whilst they were still in the closet. That is, they experienced gender phenomenology of the appropriate type even before they were out of the closet. Meanwhile, shifters (who describe their gender identity as having changed) tend not to describe such phenomenology.

This account isn't perfect though. One problem it faces is that of categorising gender phenomenology. In this account, having a male gender identity consists in having male gender phenomenology, having a female gender identity consists in having female gender phenomenology, having a nonbinary gender identity consists in having nonbinary gender phenomenology, and so on for all the other genders. But if that's right, then we need some way of sorting gender phenomenology into male, female, nonbinary, and other categories. Some phenomenology might be relatively easy to categorise. The experience Chu described, for instance, of longing to be a woman, seems obviously to belong to the category of female gender phenomenology. Others, however, are less easy to categorise. Take, for example, the experience of feeling claustrophobic in a stereotypically male body. Sure, this might be female gender phenomenology, but it could also be nonbinary gender phenomenology, genderqueer phenomenology, and many other categories besides. Which one is it? Well, for Chappell, it gave rise to a female gender identity, but for many people, a feeling of claustrophobia in a stereotypically male body instead gives rise to a genderqueer gender identity. As such, we might think that we can't define gender identity in terms of gender phenomenology *alone*. We need something over and above just the gender phenomenology to give us gender identity.

Here's another reason you might be wary of the gender phenomenology as gender identity account: it seems as if it doesn't really work well for cisgender people's gender identities. Whilst most trans people experience a rich gender phenomenology, cis people are often stumped by the thought that there is something that it is like to be (say) a woman, at least in the sense that we're discussing here. Julia Serano has suggested that this "blind spot" when it comes to gender phenomenology arises from the fact that cisgender people's gender identities, their bodies, and their social genders all seem to line up nicely and that it is only the friction caused by a mismatch here that leads to the experience of gender phenomenology.[12] Regardless of the precise reason that many cisgender people lack the experiences of gender phenomenology as described by transgender people, it's clear that such a lack causes issues for the gender identity as gender phenomenology account. Why? Well, think about what the account has to say about such people: if gender identity just is gender phenomenology, then such cisgender people don't have gender identities.

Is this such a bad result? Well, it is pretty counterintuitive: most men come out as not having male gender identities in this account! Another reason to think that this isn't a desirable result for a theory of gender identity also comes from Serano. She draws an analogy between gender identity and sexual orientation. Serano says that an important part of the success of gay, lesbian, and bisexual activism over the past 50 years has been maintaining that all people have a sexual orientation. That is, rather than treating gay people as aberrations from natural sexuality, queer activists have argued that everyone has a sexual orientation – straight people included. This sort of move seems to undermine certain forms of homophobia by insisting that (in an important sense) lesbians, gay men, and bisexual people are *just like* straight people. For Serano, a similar move should be made with gender identity if transgender activism is to have the same kind of success as lesbian, gay, and bisexual activism. We shouldn't say that trans people are radically different from cis people because trans people have a gender identity where cis people don't. Instead, suggests Serano, we should insist that everyone has a gender identity. It's just that cisgender people's gender identities match the gender that they were assigned at birth, whereas transgender people's gender identities don't![13]

MAKING SENSE

It seems as if gender phenomenology is something important that we should make sense of in thinking about gender identity. But we need something more than an account that just reduces gender identity to gender phenomenology. One option here is to include room for our interpretations of the gender phenomenology that we experience. So, our gender identity isn't the gender phenomenology itself but rather how we make sense of those experiences. I argue for a position that says gender identity is just our beliefs about what our gender is.[14] Our gender phenomenology (among other things) can cause us to have this or that belief about what gender(s) we are, but in this account, the gender identity is just those beliefs. If you believe that you're nonbinary, then you have a nonbinary gender identity, if you believe that you're a man, then you have a male gender identity. I call this type of theory of gender identity a 'deflationary' account of gender identity, because it deflates the sort of thing that a gender identity is: all there is to having a gender identity is having a belief of a particular sort.

This kind of deflationary account of gender identity has several nice features. For one, it's very simple, and seems to get everyone's gender identity 'right'. Even cis people (who seemed to pose a problem for gender identity as gender phenomenology) still have beliefs about what gender they are. As such, the vast majority of people will have a gender identity in this account. Moreover, there's no problem of having to categorise the gender phenomenology: each person interprets their own gender phenomenology for themselves, and comes to their own beliefs about what gender they are.

There is, however, something of a gap in the picture here. How do we come to these beliefs about our genders? Sure, our gender phenomenology (in some way, partly) causes those beliefs, but the deflationary account doesn't do much to illustrate exactly what's going on here. Now, there's surely a lot of variety in this context: Nicholas and Chu, for example, seemed to form beliefs about their genders via very different routes. As such, it looks like it's going to be difficult to give a universal story about the process here – and perhaps we shouldn't! It would still be nice, however, if we could give at least some gestures towards some of the processes that are often involved in forming beliefs about our genders.

Florence Ashley approaches this task using a couple of metaphors for construction. For Ashley, our beliefs about our genders can be understood as attempts to construct a story that explains (a part of) who we are. We try to understand why we have certain gender phenomenology, how we are treated as we move through the world, our relation to gender norms, and so on. Making sense of a life in this way, they suggest, often involves building a narrative about who we are. Part of this narrative construction involves adopting beliefs about what's going on and who we are, including beliefs about our gender(s), that make the story fit together.

So, suppose that you were assigned female at birth and have been raised as a girl. Yet you've felt deeply uncomfortable in your body and felt a deep longing to take on a more masculine body. One possible way of making sense of these experiences is by thinking that you're a trans man. Certainly, the narrative of your life makes sense read through this lens. This is not, however, the only way that you could build a belief about your gender out of these experiences. You might instead begin to think of yourself as genderqueer, as a transmasc nonbinary person, as a cisgender woman who feels discomfort with her body, or as something else entirely!

Ashley uses a different construction metaphor to explore this idea:

> For the same gender subjectivity, different architects will select different columns as load-bearing based on personal predispositions. Whereas some trans people link their gender identity to bodily discomfort and dysphoria, others do not experience gender dysphoria nor desire medical transition. Though there may be no hard and fast rules, I suggest that affect in relation to gender categorization, belonging-with, gender labels, and pronouns, as well as experiences of gender euphoria and gender dysphoria, are often load-bearing among trans people, playing a central role in the constitution of gender identity, whereas external gender categorization, gendering of the body, and the application of gender norms are more often load-bearing among cis people.[15]

Is this the right account? Well, you might worry that the process being described here is too intentional. That is, it looks like a creative and reflective practice that takes time and intent to achieve. Whilst this kind of activity may be common among some trans people, most people don't reflect so carefully on their gender phenomenology before forming a belief about their gender: they just believe that they're a woman or believe that they're a man.

However, we don't have to think that this construction process is always so conscious and detailed. Presumably it can also take place pre-reflectively or through processes of socialisation. Suppose, for instance, you were raised as a boy, were always told that you are going to become a man and chastised whenever you did something feminine. Making sense of these experiences needn't involve a conscious reflection upon them and a careful process of thinking through which gender you are to make sense of these experiences. No, you might just assume that you're a man! The belief here is formed without reflection and fits neatly with the way the world treats you – no self-conscious narrative construction required.

That's not to say that this kind of account is without its challenges. For one, you might think that the account somehow gets things the wrong way around: in this kind of account, someone has a genderqueer gender identity because they believe that they are genderqueer. But shouldn't things be the other way around? Surely, if things are going right, this person should believe that they are genderqueer because they have a genderqueer gender identity. Another challenge comes from the apparent 'shallowness' of belief. Part of what motivated our initial essentialist account of gender identity was the thought that there was something 'deep' about gender identity. That is, it is a part of who we authentically are, deep down. Beliefs, meanwhile, seem pretty easy to come by. We form and lose them all the time. According to Ashley, beliefs about our genders are even less essential than on the normal picture of beliefs: they are posits, suppositions to make narrative sense of our experience. So, if one is a deflationist about gender identity, then it looks like one is going to have to reject the thought that gender identities are deep in the sense that motivated essentialism.

GENDER AND GENDER IDENTITY

In the first chapter, we looked at gender as a social phenomenon. We thought about how people get constructed as members of particular genders, and how this process is related to things like social structures and gender norms. In this chapter, we've thought about gender as identity, thinking about the internal features of people that constitute gender identifications. But what is gender *really*? Which one of these senses of 'gender' should we privilege as gender proper?

Rach Cosker-Rowland has explored several possibilities here.[16] One option that is widely assumed in transgender circles, Cosker-Rowland calls a 'gender identity first' position. According to gender identity first accounts, gender is really just gender identity. Gender as social role or conferred property are interesting features of the world, but they aren't gender proper: gender identity is what gender really is. This kind of position has some nice upshots. It means that when someone says that a trans woman isn't a woman, they aren't just saying something morally wrong that misgenders the trans woman, they're also saying something literally false. Moreover, the person who tries to undermine trans people by saying that they are mistaken about their genders also turns out to have just misunderstood what gender really is.

This account runs into a few challenges, though. One comes from thinking about people who lack gender identities. Elizabeth Barnes raises the example of people whose cognitive impairment means that they cannot form beliefs of the form 'I am a woman'. It looks like the gender identity first account is forced to say that such people don't have gender identities, and therefore they don't have genders, really. But this seems like a troubling conclusion. For one, Barnes suggests that this reinforces the ostracisation and othering of disabled people by treating them as akin to animals. After all, we also refrain from gendering many critters, especially things like insects. It seems morally troubling to have a position that treats disabled people as like insects! Another issue is that there seem to be important features of such cognitively disabled people's experience that need to be seen through a gendered lens, not least the sexual violence faced by many disabled women. By suggesting that such people aren't 'really' women, we might wonder whether this sort of account impoverishes our understanding of the specific forms that violence against such people takes.[17]

Another option Cosker-Rowland considers is that some of the senses considered previously, when taken together, are gender proper. Here the idea might be that both gender identity and gender as social role are gender – something suggested by Katharine Jenkins.[18] Let's call this kind of thing a 'dual' theory of gender. How is a dual theory of gender supposed to work? Well, in the case where you are a man according to both gender identity and social role, the dual account will say that you are a man in the real or proper sense of gender. Meanwhile if you aren't a man according to both, then you aren't a man, full stop. However, what if the two senses of gender disagree? What if you have a male gender identity but a female social role, or vice versa? One option would be to privilege one sense of gender over the other: that when the two conflict, (say) gender as identity takes priority. But this seems undermotivated: why think that one sense takes priority over others?

One option might be to prioritise one sense of gender over the others on moral, pragmatic, and political grounds. Take, for example, Sam. Suppose that Sam is a wealthy, powerful, and high-flying businessperson, and also identifies as a trans woman, although she isn't out to most people yet. One might think that Sam, because she isn't out, will count as a man according to those senses of 'gender' which analyse gender solely in terms of the kind of position that someone has in society or how one is treated interpersonally. However, on gender identity senses of 'gender' she will count as a woman because she identifies as a woman. Nevertheless, we might think that we have good moral reason to privilege gender as identity here: after all, we'd be misgendering her if we treated her as a man when she has a female gender identity.

However, why should these moral reasons for treating Sam this way tell us anything about what the world is in fact like? That is, we were trying to figure out the truth of gender 'really' is, not what would be the best way to act. To assume that the facts about the world match onto how we should act so neatly seems like wishful thinking.

There are other possibilities that one might adopt in figuring out what gender 'really' is. However, there is a different approach that we might take here, including drawing on the pluralist approaches we encountered in the last chapter. That is, we can challenge the thought that there must be a thing which is 'really' gender. According to this view, there's no one sense of 'gender' that the world privileges as gender proper. There's gender identity, gender as social role, gendered social structures, gender as conferred property, and more besides. All these things are gender, and none is privileged as the 'real' thing. When we say "Charlie is a man" we could be saying that Charlie has a male gender identity or that Charlie has been conferred the property of being a man by his community. We just need to be clearer about which sense of these gender terms that we're using!

Now, suppose one agrees with this thought, that there's nothing out there in the world that privileges one sense of gender over others. That doesn't mean that one has to be neutral about which sense we should in fact use. As explored previously, there are often good moral, political, and pragmatic reasons to prefer usage that matches certain senses rather than others. As such, we have moral reason to prefer gender identity uses of gender over certain social structure uses in certain contexts, and reason to prefer other senses in other contexts. Unlike the dual theory of gender, this position doesn't fall victim to claims of wishful thinking. Why? Because it doesn't claim that this or that sense of gender is 'really' gender. Instead, it just says that there are different ways that we should act towards one another.

In the next chapter we'll think carefully about this 'should': what kind of justification is provided to you when I say, "I am agender"? Should you treat me as agender because it would be morally wrong to do otherwise, or because it's the truth?

NOTES

1 NHS. (2022). "Gender Identity", in *Data Quality of Protected Characteristics and Other Vulnerable Groups*. https://digital.nhs.uk/data-and-information/data-collections-and-data-sets/data-sets/mental-health-services-data-set/submit-data/data-quality-of-protected-characteristics-and-other-vulnerable-groups/gender-identity (accessed 09 January 2024).

2 Nagel, Thomas. (1979). "What it is Like to Be a Bat?". *Philosophical Review* 83(4): 430–450.

3 Chappell, Sophie-Grace. (2025). *Trans Figured: On Being a Transgender Person in a Cisgender World*. Bristol: Polity, §1.14.
4 Benjamin, Harry. (1966/1999). *The Transsexual Phenomenon*. Düsseldorf: Symposium.
5 Benjamin, *The Transsexual Phenomenon*, 110, 140.
6 Pearce, Ruth. (2018). *Understanding Trans Health: Discourse, Power and Possibility*. Bristol: Polity, pp. 33–36.
7 Prosser, Jay. (1998). *Second Skins: The Body Narratives of Transsexuality*. New York: Columbia University Press, p. 69.
8 Nicholas, Harry. (2023). *A Trans Man Walks into a Gay Bar: A Journey of Self (and Sexual) Discovery*. London and Philadelphia: Jessica Kingsley, pp. 35–36.
9 Chu, Andrea Long. (2019). *Females*. London and New York: Verso, p. 79.
10 Talusan, Meredith, Tobia, Jacob, Milan, Tiq and Nico, Fonseca. (2016). "Telling Trans Stories Beyond 'Born in the Wrong Body". *Buzzfeed.com*. https://www.buzzfeed.com/meredithtalusan/telling-trans-stories-beyond-born-in-the-wrong-body
11 Cull, Matthew J. (2024c). *What Gender Should Be*. London: Bloomsbury, pp. 115–116.
12 Serano, Julia. (2016). *Whipping Girl: A Transsexual Woman on Sexism and the Scapegoating of Femininity*, 2nd edn. Berkeley: Seal Press, p. 87.
13 Serano, *Whipping Girl*, 89.
14 Cull, *What Gender Should Be*, 117–119.
15 Ashley, Florence. (2023). "What is it Like to Have a Gender Identity?". *Mind* 132(528): 1062.
16 Cosker-Rowland, Rach. (2023). "Recent Work on Gender Identity and Gender". *Analysis* 83(4): 801–820.
17 Barnes, Elizabeth. (2019). "Gender and Gender Terms". *Noûs* 54(3): 704–730.
18 Jenkins, Katharine. (2016). "Amelioration and Inclusion: Gender Identity and the Concept of Woman". *Ethics* 126(2): 403–404.

RECOMMENDATIONS FOR FURTHER READING

In addition to the works already cited in this chapter, some works that have been important philosophical contributions to the study of gender identity include:

B.R. George and R.A. Brigg's "Science Fiction Double Feature" is a rich and philosophically intriguing exploration of how we might make sense of gender, gender phenomenology, and gender identity. This discussion is deepened in their recent book, *What Even Is Gender?*

Briggs, R.A. and George, B.R. (2023). *What Even Is Gender?*. Abingdon and New York: Routledge.

George, B.R. and Briggs, R.A. (unpublished). "Science Fiction Double Feature: Trans Liberation on Twin Earth". https://philpapers.org/archive/GEOSFD.pdf

Jennifer Saul's 2012 paper provides some of the first exploration of the sorts of objections that we levelled at the deflationary account:

Saul, Jennifer. (2012). "Politically Significant Terms and Philosophy of Language: Methodological Issues", in Sharon Crasnow and Anita Superson (eds.) *Out from the Shadows: Analytical Feminist Contributions to Traditional Philosophy*. Oxford: Oxford University Press.

Katharine Jenkins' work provides an account of gender identity as a set of 'maps', and provides the dual theory of gender used as a foil by Cosker-Rowland. More recently she has moved away from this position to a version of pluralism, as discussed in Chapter 1, though her 2018 paper develops the map idea further:

Jenkins, Katharine. (2018). "Toward an Account of Gender Identity". *Ergo* 5(27). https://doi.org/10.3998/ergo.12405314.0005.027

Elizabeth Barnes' work on cognitive disability has provided an important challenge to gender identity first accounts. She explores these ideas more fully in her 2022 paper:

Barnes, Elizabeth. (2022). "Gender Without Gender Identity: The Case of Cognitive Disability". *Mind* 131(523): 836–862.

An interesting account of gender as gender identity that relies on dispositions, rather than beliefs, hence straddling both internal and external aspect of gender is given by Jennifer McKitrick:

McKitrick, Jennifer. (2015). "A Dispositional Account of Gender". *Philosophical Studies* 172(10): 2575–2589.

Rach Cosker-Rowland has recently developed a sophisticated view of gender as 'fittingness' drawing on her work in metaethics:

Cosker-Rowland, Rach. (2025). *Gender Identity: What it is and Why it Matters.* Oxford: Oxford University Press.

E.M Hernandez and Rowan Bell put forward another deflationary account of gender identity:

Hernandez, E.M. and Bell, Rowan. (2025). "Much Ado About Nothing: Unmotivating 'Gender Identity'". *Ergo: An Open Access Journal of Philosophy* 12(50): 1313–1340.

3

KNOWLEDGE AND JUSTIFICATION

Imagine that you have a friend named George. George has a male gender identity, and says things like "I'm a man," and "Please use the pronouns he/him/his when referring to me." Now (barring odd circumstances) you'd be right to think that you are *justified* in believing that George is a man and that you would be *justified* in acting in ways that treat George as a man. But what is the nature of this justification? That is, why are you right to believe that George is a man, and why are you right to act in ways that treat George as a man?

One answer that you might give to these questions is that you are justified in acting and believing this way because it's *true*. This would be an *epistemic* justification. Another answer that you might give is that you are justified in acting and believing this way because, *morally* speaking, it's the right thing to do and believe. This would be an *ethical* justification. But, which of these is answers is right? Are we right to believe that George is a man because it is true that he's a man or because it's the ethical thing to believe? Are we right in acting towards George in ways that treat him as a man because it's true that he's a man, or because it's the ethical thing to do?

DOI: 10.4324/9781003502944-4

ETHICS AND EPISTEMOLOGY

You will probably have come across the term 'ethics' before. As we'll think about it here, it's the study of things like what is morally right and wrong, and what makes something good and bad. Ethics asks questions like "is it always wrong to lie?" and "why is lying acceptable in certain circumstances?" An ethicist might say that, whilst lying is usually bad, it's occasionally the right thing to do. A classic example here is the case of an axe murderer at the door: suppose you are hiding a friend from someone who wants to murder her, and then the murderer knocks at the door and asks you where your friend is. Here, most people agree that it's okay to lie to the murderer! But why is it okay to lie in this circumstance, but not most other circumstances? Ethicists have a variety of preferred answers to this question. One ethical justification for lying to the murderer at the door might be this: we should always act as to minimise the total amount of harm to others and ourselves. Generally, lying does more harm than good, so we aren't justified in lying most of the time. However, in the murderer at the door case, we are justified in lying because the harm we do to the murderer in lying to them is outweighed by the harm that would result from us telling the truth. The disrespect and betrayal that the murderer might feel after they find out we have lied to them is nowhere near as bad as our friend being killed by an axe-wielding murderer!

Different ethicists tend to appeal to different things when talking about ethical justification. Some appeal to things like maximising everyone's happiness, or minimising pain. Others appeal to the rights of individuals and groups – so something would be wrong *because* it violates someone's rights. Still others talk in terms of virtue, others the value of caring, and so on. We don't have to make up our minds as to which of these groups of ethicists is right here! Crucial here, however, is recognising that they are offering different explanations of what makes things good and bad, morally right and morally wrong.

Moral rightness and wrongness aren't the only types of rightness and wrongness though. Suppose you and I are playing a maths game, and you challenge me tell you what the square root of 81 is. I answer 8, sincerely believing it to be the right answer. Now, it's clear that I've got this wrong. After all, $\sqrt{81} = 9$, not 8. However, whilst it's clear that I've got the answer wrong, and I have definitely done something wrong in my calculation, I've not done anything *morally* wrong. Instead, I'm wrong here because I've said something *false*.

It's less likely that you'll have heard of 'epistemology' than ethics. For our purposes here, we can think of it as the field that studies why we are justified or unjustified in cases like this, where truth and falsity are at issue. It also studies the nature of knowledge and evidence, and alongside questions of expertise and disagreement.

Let's take a different example. Suppose you and I have been in a basement for the past six hours, talking about trans philosophy. Because this basement is deep underground, there aren't any windows, and so we can't see what the weather is like outside. Worried about our respective journeys home, we begin to wonder whether it will rain. You say, "I believe that it will rain" and put on your coat, and I do the same. However, whilst we both agree on what to believe and what to do, our justifications are different. You base your belief that it's raining on the weather forecast that you just looked up on your phone's weather app. Meanwhile, I base my belief that it's raining on the tea leaves in my mug: I think that I can tell the future by reading them! The purported justifications for our beliefs and actions here are both *epistemic*: it's not a question of whether either of us is doing something morally wrong in believing that it will rain and putting on a coat. Rather, we have both gone through some process of trying to find out about what the world is like, and the question is whether such processes get us to the truth or not. Of course, your process is a lot better than mine! Weather forecasts aren't perfect, but they are generally reliable, especially about the near future. By contrast, reading tea leaves to divine the future is complete bunk! Indeed, you might think that because reading tea leaves is so unreliable, I am not justified in believing that it will rain at all!

Let's return to the question that set off this discussion of the difference between ethical and epistemic justification. George identifies as a man, and we take ourselves to be justified in treating him as a man, and justified in believing that he is a man. However, is this justification more like the justification for lying to the axe-murderer or your justification for thinking that it will rain? Should we act this way towards George and believe that he is a man because it is ethically the right thing to do or because it is epistemically the right thing to do?

BETTCHER'S CHALLENGE TO EPISTEMIC FIRST-PERSON AUTHORITY

One thing you might say here is this: George said he's a man, and if anyone is an expert on George's gender identity, it's George! He's in a better position to know about his gender identity than anyone else. By virtue of being George, he has a special status that means we should trust his opinion on anything going on in George's head. He has *epistemic* first-person authority. Just as we should trust meteorologists to tell us about the weather ahead of those who read tea leaves, George is an expert on his gender identity. As such, our justification for believing George is epistemic.

However, Talia Mae Bettcher has put pressure on epistemic justifications in this context. Why? In short, because we can be wrong about what's going on in our heads. For example, sometimes when I'm feeling down, I eat too much ice cream, even though I'm full, and feel sick afterwards. During one of these sad periods, you might ask me whether I want more ice cream, and I would say "Yes, I would love more ice cream!" But of course, I'm wrong: I don't want more ice cream; it will make me sick; I am just sad. So, sometimes we can be wrong about what we want or believe! This isn't the only kind of self-deception that exists of course: denial, wishful thinking, unconscious attitudes, and all sorts of other psychological phenomena show that we are not always right about the things that go on in our heads.[1]

If we can be so drastically wrong about our inner lives, this puts pressure on the idea that we are experts or epistemic authorities about them. After all, someone who keeps getting things wrong about some topic should hardly be counted as an expert on that topic! And if we're not experts about things like our gender identities, it seems hard to see what epistemic justification could be had here.

With that said, you might think that this is a little too quick. One argument that I've made against Bettcher on this point relies on the idea that we don't always require that someone is an expert on something that they talk about before we believe them. Most of the time, we just require that they have some evidence on the matter at hand.[2] Let's return to the weather example from the start of this chapter: suppose that shortly after consulting tea leaves and the weather forecast, our friend descends the stairs to our windowless basement and says that the weather is beautiful outside, with clear skies from horizon to horizon. It's not going to rain! Now, our friend is not an expert: they don't have a PhD in meteorology. But, they do have evidence that we don't have: they were just outside looking at the weather. Here, we have good (epistemic) justification to change our beliefs about what the weather will look like.

So, sometimes at least, we don't need expertise in order to be epistemically justified in believing someone about this or that issue. We just need to recognise that they are in a better position to know about that issue or have access to evidence that we don't have. In the case of gender identity, it looks like this condition is met: only I have access to my inner life via introspection, so I have evidence about my gender identity that you don't have. Of course, sometimes this evidence is undermined by things like self-deception and denial. As such, we are not *always* epistemically justified in trusting someone's claim that they have this or that gender identity. However, generally we need some further reason to think that some person is in a condition of self-deception or denial before we start distrusting them on these issues. In general, we might think, epistemic justification is provided by individuals reporting what they think or feel.

OVERALL'S CHALLENGE TO EPISTEMIC FIRST-PERSON AUTHORITY

A different kind of challenge to epistemic justification comes from Christine Overall. Whereas Bettcher was concerned about introspection in general, Overall is worried specifically about the content of gendered experiences. She argues that it is unclear that certain experiences can straightforwardly justify claims like 'I am a woman'. Epistemic authority, says Overall, cannot come from "direct awareness of a datum".[3]

How is this argument supposed to work? Let's think first about the general narrative that many people tell about trans experiences. The story goes like this: before they realise that they are trans, the trans person goes through a range of odd phenomenology or experiences, perhaps including a rejection of the gender norms imposed upon them, a desire to have a different kind of body, or a feeling of affinity for a gender other than the one that they were assigned at birth. The story continues that this phenomenology is recognised as showing the person in question that they are not a member of the gender that they were assigned at birth.

Take the case of a trans woman called Simone, who, before she realises that she is trans, experiences precisely those kinds of phenomenology: she rejects the gender norms associated with manhood, wants to have a feminine body, and finds herself feeling a great affinity with the women in her life. She concludes that, because she is experiencing these things, she must really be a woman.

Overall's worry is that there is nothing about the phenomenology that Simone experiences that directly justifies the conclusion that Simone is a woman. After all, it is quite compatible with experiencing those things that Simone instead conclude that she is a man or nonbinary person who rejects male gender norms, wants to have a feminine body, and feels an affinity with the women in her life. This is supported by the way that confusion and doubt often accompany such experiences. It is not always clear what this or that experience means for who we are, and it's not as if there's some phenomenology that just self-evidently presents itself as women's phenomenology or womanly phenomenology! Another way of putting this, which we mentioned in the previous chapter, is that there is no way of neatly splitting up gender phenomenology into male, female, agender, and other categories. The phenomenology itself cannot determine which gender identity a person has.

Does this mean we have to give up on any sort of epistemic authority when it comes to gender identifications? Overall thinks not. She suggests that rather than being read directly off gender phenomenology, our gender identifications are interpretations of that phenomenology. The feelings of doubt and puzzlement that arise from seemingly odd aspects of our experience call us to try to make sense of our phenomenology. So, for Overall, there's a step missing in the story that we told about Simone previously: one in which Simone uses the concepts and understandings of gender that she has inherited from her society in order to make sense of her experiences. Much like Ashley and myself, whose views on gender identity we discussed in the last chapter, Overall claims that our gender identities are interpretative constructions that we use to make sense of the continuing narratives of our lives.

You might wonder whether this is enough to give us epistemic authority regarding our gender identities. After all, if our gender identities are just interpretations of some phenomenology, it's perfectly possible for there to be other interpretations of that phenomenology. And who's to say which interpretation is the best one? Think of novels: these have multiple interpretations, and it's unclear as to how to adjudicate which is the best or most authoritative interpretation. Indeed, following the arguments of Roland Barthes, it is now a commonplace assumption that even the author's own interpretation of the text is not automatically the correct one.[4]

Now, one thing we might say here is that one person does have something of a privileged position with respect to the gender phenomenology: the person experiencing it has a much more direct experience of what it is like! Unlike a novel, in the case of constructing gender identity, it is not just that the author is a particularly important interpreter because they construct the narrative. Rather, the person having the phenomenology has access to data that the 'reader' doesn't.

EPISTEMIC INJUSTICE AND ETHICAL FIRST-PERSON AUTHORITY

Regardless of whether one buys the previous arguments for or against epistemic first-person authority, it seems clear that we (also) have some sort of *ethical* duty to act towards others in ways that are justified by their gender identifications. That is, we would be doing something morally wrong if we misgendered someone. But what exactly is wrong with misgendering someone?

Being misgendered often feels like an insult. Even when it's not done on purpose, it can feel like the person doing the misgendering has snubbed you, or not taken the time to think about how their actions might impact you. This can have serious psychological impacts, especially if the misgendering happens regularly.[5] Being misgendered is linked to experiences of depression, stress, feelings of being stigmatised, and other forms of psychological distress. In short, misgendering appears to cause real psychological harm. If we think that we have a moral duty to avoid causing unnecessary harm, then we should probably conclude that we have an ethical duty to act in ways that treat a person as the gender as the gender they claim to be.

Some philosophers have explored further ways that misgendering might be morally problematic. Stephanie Kapusta has explored the idea that misgendering involves a kind of epistemic injustice that Miranda Fricker has called 'hermeneutical injustice'. *Epistemic* injustices are cases of injustice that importantly involve doing wrong to someone in their capacity as a knower. What does this mean? Well, take for example, silencing. Silencing can be seen as an epistemic injustice: by silencing you I prevent you from sharing the things that you know, and devalue you as a source of knowledge or as someone whose perspective matters. *Hermeneutical* injustices are another type of epistemic injustice. These involve preventing people from having the language or concepts to understand their own experience, and from being able to share that understanding of their experience with wider society.[6]

Kapusta argues that trans people are prevented from being able to shape the concepts of gender that society uses by virtue of being misgendered. She writes,

> Transgender persons are denied the discursive resources to participate in furthering society's understanding of their own gender and – I would add – of gender more generally. By being persistently classified as a "man" according to particular conceptions and descriptions, a transgender woman is denied participation in shaping those descriptions herself.[7]

So, for Kapusta, if you're a nonbinary person who is being misgendered all the time, you will have little opportunity to shape how society views nonbinary people. After all, if no one recognises that you're nonbinary, no one will recognise the things you do as 'what a nonbinary person does'! This means that it's only others who will define what the nonbinary experience is like. Kapusta characterises this as robbing trans people of the "power to express their own senses of self, and of the opportunity to develop a language and conceptual resources that articulate those senses of self".[8]

Of course, we might think that this isn't entirely right: surely there's little stopping a trans person from developing new ways of thinking and talking about their gender, even if they're being misgendered. And even people who aren't a part of some gender can shape how society thinks about that gender. Certainly, it looks like men have often had a powerful (and troubling) role in shaping everyone's understanding of women and women's roles in society, arguing that (for example) women's place is in the kitchen! However, unlike in the case of male domination, it's unclear how much power trans people have to be able to contribute to ways of thinking about gender in society at large, let alone enforce their ways of thinking about their own genders on the whole of society. Men, by contrast, have been able to dominate conversations on what a woman is and should be for centuries! So perhaps the hermeneutical injustice going on here is about this power imbalance: of who has the power to contribute to shift mainstream understandings of gender. It certainly looks like trans people (largely) lack this power whilst cisgender men (largely) have it due to centuries of patriarchal rule.

Another type of epistemic injustice is *testimonial* injustice. Testimonial injustice involves wrongly treating someone as not a credible source of knowledge because of some prejudice. Think, for example, of a racist patient who, because their doctor is Black, doesn't believe the doctor when she says, "You have cancer". The patient instead demands a second opinion from a White doctor, and only when the White doctor confirms the diagnosis does the patient believe it. This is a clear case of racist testimonial injustice: the Black doctor is an expert in medicine, and the patient wrongly treats her as an uncredible source because of her race. As such, there is a moral wrong done to the Black doctor – she has been wronged in her capacity as a knower.

You might think a similar thing goes on when people don't believe trans people's gender self-identifications. Trans people, you might think, are the experts on their own gender identities! Or, given the discussion earlier in this chapter, they are at very least generally in a better position than those around them to understand their own gender identities. If I tell you sincerely that I'm nonbinary, you should probably believe me, because I'm a credible source of knowledge on my own gender identity. But of course, many trans people aren't believed when they assert their gender identities. Instead, they are often treated as either lying, misguided, or delusional. You might think that this is a case of testimonial injustice: people are not giving trans people the appropriate amount of credibility because of a prejudice.[9]

So here too, we might claim, we have an ethical justification for believing people when they make a sincere claim about their own gender: because to disbelieve them would be an injustice. However, note something interesting about this kind of ethical justification: it relies on there being an epistemic justification for believing gender identity claims. Why? Because in order for there to be an injustice, the credibility we assign to an individual when they make some utterance has to be wrongly lowered due to prejudice – like racism lowering someone's confidence in a Black doctor. But if the credibility that we *should* assign is low because of non-prejudicial reasons – like not trusting someone without medical training to diagnose you with cancer – then there isn't an injustice. You're just assigning them the right level of credibility! So, if self-deception and denial do in fact undermine self-knowledge, then lowering our credence in statements about mental states is not prejudicial: it's just the correct way to assess the reliability of that person's testimony. If that's right, then thinking that we are not justified in believing gender identity claims is not a testimonial injustice.

Where does that leave us? Well, it looks as if trying to base ethical first-person authority on claims about testimonial injustice relies on the sorts of consideration that we were also concerned about when it came to *epistemic* first-person authority: the reliability of knowledge about our own mental states. So, it looks as if this kind of testimonial injustice basis for ethical first-person authority is inseparable from epistemic first-person authority. Of course, this doesn't tell us that there isn't ethical first-person authority: one might think that denial and self-deception aren't enough to undermine us as reliable witnesses about our own mental states. Or, one might try to find a different way to justify ethical first-person authority, perhaps using Kapusta's work on hermeneutical injustice, claims about the psychological harms of misgendering, or another framework entirely.

BETTCHER ON ETHICAL FIRST-PERSON AUTHORITY

Bettcher offers a further different framework for thinking about ethical first-person authority; one that doesn't rely on considerations surrounding epistemic injustice. Bettcher begins from thinking about how we treat and share with one another in intimate ways, and how such sharing can make us vulnerable to one another. Important to this kind of intimate relationship with others is the idea that we can have boundaries that delineate private parts of ourselves from more generally publicly accessible parts of ourselves. Having such boundaries enables us to be intimate with others by lifting those boundaries. For example, by sharing private thoughts and feelings with someone close. If I want to indicate to you that I think you are one of my closest friends, I might share with you an intimate and embarrassing part of my history, letting you into that small circle of people that know I was a fan of the band Fall Out Boy.

Such intentional lifting of one's boundaries is an important capacity, one that is necessary for certain forms of intimacy. Suppose, for instance, that you and I have grown closer and closer over the years, and I finally reveal to you that I am gay. My revealing of this aspect of myself to you might demonstrate my trust in you, that I feel comfortable around you, or that your importance to me demands that I share this private aspect of myself. My coming out to you here is a form of intimacy, one that I choose to engage in by asserting my boundaries and telling you that you are welcome inside them.

Contrast this case with someone who finds out about my sexuality through some other means, perhaps through seeing me in a compromising moment, and then tells you that I am gay. There's much that's morally troubling about this kind of case, not least the nonconsensual voyeurism. However, Bettcher wants to draw our attention to the idea that in revealing my sexuality to you, this third party has removed my ability to be intimate with you by sharing my sexuality with you myself. If you already know that I'm gay, I can't welcome you into the circle of those who know this about me through an intimate act of sharing. My privacy has already been violated, my boundary opened up to you without my consent, and I can no longer be intimate in this way with you. As Bettcher puts it,

> Self-display is fundamental in that it is linked to the nature of the interpersonal object as a boundaried being in a way that other intimate gestures are not. For instance, the very wrongness of violating an object's boundary derives from the fact that undermining it undermines an object's capacity to engage in self-display and therefore the capacity to reveal itself as an agent, and therefore to engaging in any gesture of intrinsic intimacy.[10]

Similarly, we might think that someone saying "I am non-binary" can be construed as a form of intimacy: a sharing of some private aspect of themself. Someone 'outing' this person as non-binary thus denies them an important capacity for intimacy.

So far, Bettcher has provided us with a nice argument against non-consensual outing, in that such outing prevents us from being able to engage in an important form of interpersonal intimacy. However, you might think that this doesn't give us an argument for first-person authority, or indeed an argument against misgendering. After all, suppose you are non-binary, and I go around misgendering you by telling people that you are a trans woman. Here I have not removed your capacity for intimate sharing of your actual gender identity with others, precisely *because* I've misgendered you. Should you choose, you can still come out to the people I was talking to. Nor can Bettcher appeal to a right to privacy over your internal mental states here. Because I've very much *not* revealed your gender identity in misgendering you, I can't be said to have violated any putative right to your privacy.[11]

Can Bettcher's argument here be adapted to tell us what is going wrong in the previous misgendering case? Well, we might think that there is something troubling about the notion that some person 'speaks for' another person without that other person's permission. Regardless of whether I'm right when I say, "Jennifer loves you", it seems like I'm doing something ethically troubling in purporting to speak for Jennifer about such private aspects of herself as whom she loves. Spelling out exactly what is morally wrong here looks like it might require thinking once again about epistemic injustice: questions of who gets to speak, who gets listened to, and whose ways of thinking about intimate features of our lives are taken for granted.

DOING THINGS WITH WORDS

A somewhat different approach to these sorts of question is put forward by Quill Kukla and Mark Lance. Thinking about the justification of gender ascriptions, they think that the standard model of thinking about their justification in terms of moral or epistemic justification misses something important: that gender ascriptions have a *pragmatic* function: "to organize social space, and support or undermine people's bodily agency, and self-determination within this social space".[12] This is to rethink gender ascriptions as *doing* something, rather than just saying something.

That our words can do things beyond just reporting things as true and false has been widely studied in philosophy at this point, with much work specifying different kinds of 'speech acts'. Some speech acts, like asserting, involve putting things forward as true or false. Others, like commanding, annulling, and advising, involve putting forward a decision about a course of action that is to be taken. These latter three types of speech act are types of *exercitive*. A classic example of an exercitive is an order. When the military general says to his officer, "polish your boots, colonel!" they are instituting a social norm. In this case, it's that the officer needs to get to work with a polishing kit! Another case is that of marrying. When a priest says to a (hopefully happy) couple, "I now pronounce you husband and wife", the priest makes the couple married, and in doing so makes them subject to the norms of married life. The priest's pronouncement doesn't just recognise the relationship between the couple: it makes them a married couple. This changes their social position, so that the couple must now follow all the social norms (and laws) associated with being husband and wife or face social punishment.

Kukla and Lance think that claims that are made about people's genders are exercitives. So, when someone says, "Simone is a woman", Kukla and Lance argue that this is an exercitive and hence primarily an attempt to make it such that Simone is subject to the norms that women follow and ensure that everyone treats her as a woman. We might rephrase what they are saying as something like "We should all treat Simone in ways that are appropriate for women to be treated, and she should act in ways that are appropriate for women to act. If someone fails here, they should be subject to some appropriate form of censure". Now, exactly what that treatment is, how women 'should' act, and indeed what appropriate censure is for failing to act in the right way may vary wildly between contexts. However, the important aspect of this sort of account of what is going on in gender ascription is that the speaker is putting Simone in a particular social location: that of being treated as a woman.

Of course, we can also think about the first-person case. According to this kind of account, if you say, "I am nonbinary", you are issuing an exercitive that demands that you are treated as nonbinary. We might think of it as something like a request or demand: asking others to (for example) use they/them pronouns to refer to you, with the promise that you will think worse of them or stop talking to them entirely if they fail to do so.

How does this relate to the question of justification? Well, speech acts like exercitives are justified in very different ways to speech acts like assertions. Assertions are, broadly speaking, truth-evaluable. If I make an assertion like, "the Exeter train leaves at midday", I am making a claim about how the world is, a claim that can be true or false. When asked for a justification for my assertion, I might appeal to things like "the timetable says so" or "I've seen it leave at midday all week". Such putative justifications for my assertion are epistemic in nature: they are reasons to think that what I say about the world is true.

Exercitives, by contrast, work differently. An exercitive is a speech act that is not about representing the world as it currently is. Instead, exercitives are about instituting norms for future behaviour. How then, are exercitives justified? Well, we can ask (at least) three questions: first, does the person saying the exercitive have the appropriate authority in the current social order? That is, given their social standing and the social norms that they want to institute, is it true or false that the person in question is in a position to institute those norms? Think back to our example of ordering someone to polish their boots. If the order wasn't uttered by a general to an officer, but instead by the private to a general, it won't have the appropriate authority to make anyone do anything. "Polish your boots, general!" is not an order that will have any force when given by someone of a lower rank like a private. Second, we can ask if the social norms that the exercitive is trying to put forward are ethically, pragmatically, or politically justified. Suppose the general put out this order to their soldiers midway through a battle: we might think that it's not exactly the best time to follow the order! Third, we can ask whether the social order in which the exercitive is uttered is ethically, pragmatically, or politically justified. That is, does the structure that has given this person the authority to make this utterance an ethical one? Does it serve our purposes? Does it promote injustice? In our example, we might challenge the justification of the order on the grounds that a rigid hierarchy in the military is unjust or runs into practical issues or that the existence of a military itself promotes injustice.

So, exercitives can require a variety of justifications: some epistemic, some pragmatic, some ethical, some political, and perhaps even more besides. Can we use this to think about the kinds of justification involved in gender claims? Well, let's think again about "Simone is a woman" and "I am nonbinary". We can again ask three questions about the justification of these exercitives, and in doing so, we can explore ways that gender exercitives might fail to be justified.

First, does the speaker have the appropriate authority in the current social order to make this kind of claim? In many societies, we're seeing something of a battle over who has the authority to make claims about gender. Whilst it has long been taken that individuals don't have any particularly special authority when it comes to determining their own genders, things have begun to change. As self-identification becomes more and more popular as a way of organising our gender practices, we are seeing perceptions of authority shift towards individuals. So, in a context where these sort of trans-inclusive practices are common, we might think that

"I am nonbinary" will work as an exercitive, but "Simone is a woman" may not, especially if Simone themselves expresses that they are not a woman!

Second, are the norms that this speech act puts forward ethically, politically, and pragmatically justified? Here we might ask whether it is morally appropriate to treat Simone as a woman. If Simone insisting that they are not a woman, we might think that the norms for our behaviour that "Simone is a woman" puts forward aren't justified. What about "I am nonbinary"? Here it's a little more difficult to think of an example where the exercitive may not be justified, but think of the following case: suppose you say "I am nonbinary" with the implication that I should treat you as being nonbinary all the time. However, suppose that one day we find ourselves in a context where there is the immediate threat of transphobic violence against anyone who is out as nonbinary. Here, for pragmatic reasons, it seems like we should keep your nonbinary identity hidden in order to avoid violence against you. So, at least in this context, the exercitive is not justified on pragmatic grounds.

Third, is the social order in which this speech act is uttered ethically, politically, or pragmatically justified? Here we need to assess things like whether it is politically wise for us to have the kinds of gender norms that we do. We might think, for instance, that it is politically troubling for there to be norms about what sorts of labour women should perform. As such, we might think that we need to do away with those norms if exercitives that involve ascribing womanhood are ever to be politically justified. Beyond whatever particular norms which our exercitives hold people to, we can also critically assess whether our standards for determining who has authority to make gender claims are acceptable, and even whether having gender in society is morally acceptable at all. We'll return to this last concern, about whether we should abolish gender, later in this book.

NOTES

1 Bettcher, Talia Mae. (2009). "Trans Identities and First-Person Authority", in Laurie Schrage (ed.) *You've Changed: Sex Reassignment and Personal Identity*. Oxford: Oxford University Press, pp. 98–120.

2 Cull, Matthew J. (2024b). "Un Œuf but Enough: Trans Epistemology and Methodological Radicalism". *Hypatia* 39(1): 52.

3 Overall, Christine. (2009). "Sex/Gender Transitions and Life-Changing Aspirations", in Laurie Shrage (ed.) *You've Changed: Sex Reassignment and Personal Identity*. Oxford: Oxford University Press, p. 21.
4 Barthes, Roland. (1977). "The Death of the Author", in Stephen Heath (trans.) *Image Music Text*. London: HarperCollins, pp. 142–148.
5 McLemore, K.A. (2018). "A Minority Stress Perspective on Transgender Individuals' Experiences with Misgendering". *Stigma and Health* 3(1): 53–64. https://doi.org/10.1037/sah0000070
6 Fricker, Miranda. (2007). *Epistemic Injustice: Power and the Ethics of Knowing*. Oxford: Oxford University Press.
7 Kapusta, Stephanie Julia. (2016). "Misgendering and Its Moral Contestability". *Hypatia* 31: 504. https://doi.org/10.1111/hypa.12259
8 Kapusta, "Misgendering and Its Moral Contestability".
9 Cull, Matthew J. (2022). "Epistemic Injustice and Trans Lives", in Laura Erikson-Scroth (ed.) *Trans Bodies, Trans Selves*, 2nd edn. Oxford: Oxford University Press, pp. 656–657.
10 Bettcher, Talia Mae. (2025). *Beyond Personhood: An Essay in Trans Philosophy*. Minneapolis: University of Minnesota Press, p. 46.
11 It's worth noting that Bettcher herself is mostly interested in a different kind of misgendering, *reality enforcement*, which she sees as being at the heart of much (though not all) oppression of trans people. In brief, reality enforcement is about the insistence of cisgender society that one's appearance should match the genitalia that one is supposed to have, and any failures on this front are to be policed and corrected. She provides a complex and fascinating account of the reality enforcement in *Beyond Personhood* (2025).
12 Kukla, Quill and Lance, Mark. (2022). "Telling Gender: The Pragmatics and Ethics of Gender Ascriptions". *Ergo* 9(42): 1130–1131.

RECOMMENDATIONS FOR FURTHER READING

In addition to the works already cited in this chapter, those wanting to think more about epistemology in the context of transgender philosophy might like to take a look at the following:

The best book on epistemic injustice currently on the market is by Aidan McGlynn. It's both very accessible and astonishingly comprehensive of the recent literature. I highly recommend it to anyone interested in the topic:
McGlynn, Aidan. (2026). *Epistemic Injustice: An Introduction*. New York and London: Routledge.

There have now been a few articles on the epistemic injustices faced by trans people. Three excellent examples are:
Fricker, Miranda and Jenkins, Katharine. (2017). "Epistemic Injustice, Ignorance, and Trans Experiences", in Ann Garry, Serene J. Khader, and

Alison Stone (eds.) *The Routledge Companion to Feminist Philosophy*. New York and London: Routledge, pp. 268–278.

George, B.R. and Stacey, Goguen. (2021). "Hermeneutical Backlash: Trans Youth Panics as Epistemic Injustice". *Feminist Philosophy Quarterly* 7(4).

Henckel, S.J. (2025). "You Think You Know Someone: Trans Identities and Epistemic Injustice". *Hypatia*, first look: 1–22.

Trystan Goetze has published an excellent article on hermeneutical injustices of various types and nonbinary identity:

Goetze, Trystan S. (2018). "Hermeneutical Dissent and the Species of Hermeneutical Injustice". *Hypatia* 33(1): 73–90.

Those looking to get a closer look at the epistemology of self-knowledge might like to start with the *Stanford Encyclopedia* article on the topic. Whilst it doesn't engage with trans philosophy, it is a useful collation of the broader philosophical discussion of the topic.

Gertler, Brie. (2021). "Self-Knowledge", in Edward N. Zalta (ed.) *The Stanford Encyclopedia of Philosophy* (*Winter 2021 Edition*). https://plato.stanford.edu/archives/win2021/entries/self-knowledge/

Bettcher's "Evil Deceivers and Make Believers" is a powerful exploration of the troubling stereotypes surrounding trans women as either being maliciously deceitful or as pathetically delusional.

Bettcher, Talia Mae. (2007). "Evil Deceivers and Make Believers: On Transphobic Violence and the Politics of Illusion". *Hypatia* 22(3): 43–65.

Michael Rea has developed a view on which we construct our own genders via 'self-conferral', with interesting consequences for how we think about first-person authority:

Rea, Michael. (2022). "Gender as Self-Conferred Identity". *Feminist Philosophy Quarterly* 8(2).

An exciting recent development comes from Kenneth Silver, who is interested in the broader significance of self-identification for playing a part in practices of inclusion and exclusion from groups:

Silver, Kenneth. (2026). "The Standing of Self-Identity" First View: 1–22.

4

DESIRE AND TRANSFORMATIVE EXPERIENCE

We've tried to answer a number of 'what' and 'how' questions so far in this book: What is gender? How are first person accounts of the self justified? What is gender identity? In this chapter, we'll turn to a 'why' question: why are people trans?

WHY ARE *THEY* LIKE THAT?

Being trans is, in general, not an easy form of life. Why, then, would anyone transition? The late 20th and early 21st centuries saw a few attempts to explain why trans people transition come to prominence: *biology*, *privilege*, and *fetishism*. Whilst sometimes taken up by trans people in attempting to understand themselves, it's worth noting that these purported explanations have tended to be put forward *by cisgender people*. Cis scientists, cis feminists, cis politicians, all have wanted an explanation for why trans people are different.

BIOLOGY

Biological explanations of trans people take a number of forms. However, central to such explanations is an insistence that transgender

DOI: 10.4324/9781003502944-5

people have some feature(s) of their biology that make them different from cis people, and such a difference explains why transgender people want to transition. This sort of explanation is analogous to a similar sort of explanation for queer sexual identities: that there is some gay bit of the brain, a lesbian gene, or bisexual bodily feature that means that LGBQ people were *born this way.*

One such feature that is often supposed to mark out trans people as different is their brains. That is, trans people supposedly have a brain that somehow doesn't match the rest of their body, and this explains why they want to transition. Here's how a brain-based biological explanation of trans people might go:

1. There are important differences in the brain structures between cisgender men and cisgender women.
2a. Transgender women's brain structures are closer to cisgender women's brains than they are to cisgender men's brains.
2b. Transgender men's brain structures are closer to cisgender men's brains than they are to cisgender women's brains.
2c. Non-binary people's brains comparatively do not closely resemble either those of cisgender men or women.
3. So: trans people's brains do not 'match' their bodies in the way that cis people's brains do.
4. So: trans people are caused to desire transitions so as to fix this mismatch.

Is this explanation any good? Well, one thing that we might say about this and other *born this way* explanations is that they are often politically useful. By claiming that my non-binary gender identity or my lesbian sexuality is an innate feature of my biology, I can repudiate those who would try to dismiss my gender or sexuality on the grounds that it is 'unnatural' or 'a mere choice'. In a political climate where arguments against LGBTQI+ rights are based on these sorts of grounds, a biological basis for being trans or queer might provide an important counterpoint.

However, there are a number of reasons to be sceptical of this sort of biological explanation. For one, premises 1 and 2a–2c are not obviously true. They are going to require extensive empirical investigation to figure out whether they are right or not.[1] Premise

1 is going to be especially contentious: specifying and showing the existence of such gendered brain similarities and differences across huge swathes of the varied and diverse human race is going to be extremely difficult. Moreover, it's going to be difficult to show that any systematic differences between cisgender men and cisgender women are particularly relevant to the lived experience of gendered embodiment. As such, 3 does not straightforwardly follow from 1 and 2a–2c. Why is it that having a certain similarity to cisgender men's brain structures leads to trans men to desire undertaking a gender transition? We would need more explanation than is offered here.

Finally, it's not clear that it is always a politically savvy tactic to rely on this sort of argument. After all, if we base our arguments for trans rights on the previous sort of explanation, and if it turns out that later scientific advances undermine the claim that (for instance) trans women's brains closely resemble those of cisgender women, then our argument for trans rights is undermined! Perhaps we ought to look elsewhere for our response to the person who says that transness is unnatural and thus that trans people shouldn't have the right to transition. For instance, we might instead argue that we should have the right to do plenty of things that are apparently unnatural, from wearing glasses to playing cricket!

PRIVILEGE

If biological explanations of why trans people want to transition are tendentious, perhaps it is worth looking to a social explanation instead. Maybe trans people want to transition because they see some social benefit that they can access via transition. Think, for instance, of the many benefits that can accrue to men under patriarchy – from higher wages to better healthcare due to the majority of medical research being focused on men.[2] Perhaps trans men are drawn to transition due to the attractions of such privilege: maybe they want to escape oppression as a woman.

Of course, this sort of account faces a somewhat tricky problem: why do trans women want to transition given these circumstances? If women face all sorts of oppression under patriarchy, trans women seem deeply irrational in wanting to give up the privilege of manhood for the subordination of womanhood. Those defending this sort of position have tended to suggest that trans women either sexually fetishise womanhood (we'll come back to this shortly), want to undermine the feminist movement by infiltrating it, or seek local kinds of social benefits like the supposed warmth of women's communities.[3]

There are, of course, a number of other issues with this sort of explanation of the 'why' of transition – even in explaining why trans men transition. Christine Overall notes, "trans identity, far from being a formula for privilege or protection, is in fact a marker for oppression. As Kyle Scanlon puts it, being trans means "fighting for survival, recognition, equality, housing, employment, safety and medical care"".[4] Trans men, by virtue of being trans, face oppression that offsets and undercuts many of the putative benefits they might get for being men. Take the second item in the list of advantages that many men benefit from under patriarchy from above: that men are likely to get better healthcare as the vast majority of medical research is done on men. However, most medical research is not done on *transgender* men – it's done on *cisgender* men! Trans men's bodily differences from the vast majority of other men mean that this bias in medical research won't benefit them. Indeed, there are even bigger gaps in health research on trans men than on (cisgender) women.

Meanwhile, it's hard to credit the explanations of trans women's transition here in any serious way. For one, trans women have been at the heart of a variety of feminist movements since at least the 1970s, and if they are seeking to undermine such feminisms, they are doing a spectacularly bad job.[5] Moreover, it's hard to see why one would give up a whole life of relative privilege for some local benefit like joining a local women-only space – something that not all trans women want to do in any case. The high rates of poverty, precarity, and violence faced by many trans women are crucial data point here. Transitioning does not seem like the kind of thing that one would be rationally driven to do for social benefit. Weighing up one's future life chances in society, and the degree of privilege one will have depending on whether one transitions or not: such a calculation will rarely, if ever end up favouring transition.

Are there other kinds of social privilege that might explain the desire to transition? One sort of privilege that occasionally gets suggested here is that trans people are seeking *straight privilege*. This explanation goes something like this: gay and lesbian people are subject to all sorts of oppression, violence, and subordination due to our society being homophobic and 'heteronormative', privileging straight relationships and forms of life. Being straight, and hence avoiding that oppression, violence, and subordination, is therefore a desirable privilege. As such, if you're a gay man or a lesbian, you might think that one way of accessing straight privilege is to change one's gender. After all, if you're a lesbian, and you transition genders to become a man but keep having sexual and romantic desires for women, then you are a straight man. Likewise, if you're a gay man who transitions to become a woman but continues desiring men, then you have become a straight woman. So, this story goes, we can explain the desire to transition in terms of a desire to become straight, and hence access the privileges of being straight.

There are, of course, lots of problems with this sort of explanation. For one, it doesn't explain the existence of nonbinary people at all! Crucially, it also assumes that all trans people begin life as gay men or lesbians – something that is far from true. There are also plenty of people who transition and come out as trans lesbians, or gay trans men, bisexual people, pansexual people, asexual people, and so on. It's also an explanation that can't account for many of the queer relationships *between* trans people, in what sometimes gets called 't4t'. Certainly, there are straight t4t relationships between a trans man and a trans woman, but the world of t4t relationships involves all sorts of gay, lesbian, pansexual, and polyamorous relationships among trans people.

The defender of this kind of explanation might retreat a little here, and say that they are only trying to explain the desire for transition in a small subsection of the trans population: that of gay men who transition to become straight women, and lesbians who transition to become straight men. However, this explanation *still* doesn't work even for this restricted group. For this explanation to work, it would require that straight privilege is evenly distributed. That is, that straight people are uniformly accorded privilege for being straight, and hence that anyone transitioning to being a straight person will automatically get those privileges. However, there's good reason to think that straight privilege is not evenly distributed. Being transgender, you might think, undercuts the possibility of fitting into heteronormative society. Such societies often treat straight trans people as improper or lesser versions of straight cisgender people, if they are recognised as being straight at all. In many cases, the transition won't be recognised at all, and the trans person treated as merely pretending to be a straight man or straight woman: so, they won't be extended many, if any, of the privileges of being straight.

If this kind of explanation is to work at all, we have to think that trans people don't recognise the way that coming out as trans massively undermines their position in society. But, in fact, trans people are all too aware of the dangers that transitioning can place them in, from interpersonal violence to political subordination! Nevertheless, trans people still want to transition, even in the face of the huge costs it can cause them.

FETISHISM

So, if rational calculation about social privilege will not explain why trans people want to transition, perhaps one ought to look to something *irrational* for an explanation. One sort of explanation along these lines that has been popular in certain circles in psychology suggests that trans people are being driven by a (seemingly) irrational force: sexual desire. According to psychologist Ray Blanchard, for example, trans women's desire to transition is an outgrowth of their sexual desires.

Blanchard argues that trans women who are attracted to cisgender women are *autogynephilic*. That is, they have (for whatever reason) misdirected their sexual desires that they have for women onto the idea of themselves being women. So, what motivates trans women to transition is that they have a fetish for being a woman: they get turned on by the thought of themselves wearing feminine clothes or by the thought of themselves with a vagina.[6]

This sort of explanation has been widely ridiculed, as you might expect. Julia Serano argues that one of its biggest problems is that there isn't really any good empirical evidence out there that supports it. Blanchard's early experiments have been widely critiqued, not least for failing to have a control group featuring cisgender women![7] Moreover, even if such sexual desires *were* present in trans women at rates exceeding other women, as Serano points out, it's far from clear that we can then say that those desires cause trans women to want to transition. This would be to assume causation when all we would have is correlation. Why not think instead that the causation runs the other way around and that dysphoria causes people to idealise and hence perhaps eroticise a body and form of life that they do not (yet) have?[8] Or, perhaps such sexual desires are just the result of being a woman under conditions of cisheteropatriarchy, where women, *including trans women*, are sexually objectified by an oppressive culture, and women internalise this objectifying gaze because it is constantly being shown to them in things like art and advertising.

TRANSGENDER EXPLANATIONS OF BEING TRANSGENDER

What should we say about all of this? Well, for one, the explanations on offer here don't look to be very good at all. They rely on dubious assumptions, shoddy science, and unjustified claims. Moreover, the explanations tend to contradict, or ignore entirely, the first-person accounts of what it is like to be trans. For instance, few trans women express any more sexual arousal at the thought of themselves as women than cis women do, and sexual arousal is just not what dysphoria feels like for the vast majority of trans women. Moreover, I know of few trans women who have attempted to undermine or argue against feminism: indeed, many trans women see themselves as feminists or at least in league with many feminist political projects. Moreover, the experiences, projects, and forms of life associated with being nonbinary are largely absent or an afterthought in these sorts of accounts. At best, these sorts of accounts think that what it is actually like to be trans is irrelevant to explaining why people want to transition. At worst they imply (or explicitly claim!) that trans people are deluded or deceitful, either mistaken about their experience or deliberately misleading those around them.[9]

Further, whilst maybe some of these explanations of why people are transgender come from a place of good faith and scientific curiosity, you might worry that some of these theories are developed with the aim of dismissing transition as irrational, unnatural, or bad. It would, moreover, be naïve to think that this sort of theorising happens in isolation from ongoing debates over the place of trans people in society. It certainly provides ammunition to someone seeking to remove access to gender-affirming care if that person can argue that trans people are 'just' fetishists or are trying to undermine feminism.

With these failings in mind, one thing we might try to offer is a *trans* theory of why people transition. Cisgender people have tried to give explanations of why people want to transition, but these explanations don't look very good. So, perhaps we should begin from the transgender perspectives that such explanations tend to sideline.[10]

What would such an explanation look like? Well, one explanation along these lines might appeal to so-called 'born in the wrong body' narratives. We saw something like this narrative when considering gender identity essentialism in Chapter 2. The general idea is that trans people want to transition because they are really one gender but have had the misfortune to be born in the body stereotypical of a person of some other gender. Distressed by the mismatch between their true gender and the body they have ended up with, trans people seek out transition in order to rectify this mismatch.

There are a few problems with this sort of explanation, however. What does it mean to be 'born in the wrong body'? On the one hand, one might think that this suggests something like a 'gendered soul'. Here we would posit the existence of an immaterial self that is essentially (for instance) male, which then gets born into a female body. Whilst such a set of claims might appeal to followers of certain religious traditions, this sort of reading of the 'born in the wrong body' narrative is hardly going to be convincing to everyone. On the other hand, we might suggest that the 'born in the wrong body' narrative is a claim about a mismatch between the brain and body. This would perhaps be more widely acceptable than having to admit the existence of a gendered soul! However, note that this sort of explanation seems to just be another version of the biology explanation that we considered earlier. As such, it's going to run into similar problems as that earlier account.

Moreover, it's far from clear that this explanation really is solely a *transgender* explanation of why people want to transition. The 'born in the wrong body' narrative owes no small part of its widespread cultural influence to the role it has played in gender clinics where trans people engage with medical professionals in the hope of accessing gender-affirming healthcare. Hearing a patient speak in terms of the 'born in the wrong body' narrative was often a criterion by which medical professionals could (begin to) make a diagnosis of 'transsexualism'. Ruth Pearce remarks that this kind of trans identity, then, is "constructed in *collaboration* between trans people and health professionals".[11]

Finally, whilst some trans people do think that the 'born in the wrong body' narrative gives them a good account of their own experiences of dysphoria and transition, such experiences are far from universal. Many trans people, myself included, just don't see their desire to transition or their dysphoria as fitting into this kind of narrative. This sort of consideration puts pressure on any attempt to explain *all* transness through a single explanation. The sheer variety of trans experience means that any one explanation will likely miss out on a wide array of trans people's experiences.

Perhaps then, the best we can do, in explaining the *why* of transition is something like the pluralist story that Overall puts forward, where we are complex creatures who are shaped by our society, our biology, our personal history, our economic position, ideology, our housing situation, our relationship with our mothers and so on and so forth. We are complex creatures trying to make sense of ourselves, and how we want to live going forward, often in idiosyncratic, but deeply felt ways. Sometimes, the only way to make sense of one's own particular situation is as a person who would feel more authentic, or less suicidal, or just happier, if one transitioned:

> Still, the skeptic might persist: Where do the aspirations of trans persons come from? How can they be explained? Again, my point is that aspirations for sex/gender transition are not necessarily different in kind from other deeply felt and long-held aspirations. The life-changing aspirations human beings develop and express, including the aspiration for sex/gender transition, can, I suggest, be accounted for (at least in theory, however difficult in practice that explanation may be) in terms of a mixture of personal history, social environment,

> individual interpretation, and biological factors. In some people, this network of influences contributes to a desire to be a musician; in some, they produce an eagerness to be a parent; in some, they produce spiritual aspirations; and in some, they produce an aspiration to be a person of a different sex/gender.[12]

THE POINT OF EXPLANATION

Now, a 'born in the wrong body' narrative is hardly the only available explanation for why people transition that begins from trans people and their experiences. However, at this point in the chapter, I want to ask a more fundamental question about what we are doing here. Do we need or even want an explanation for why trans people want to transition? Is this a useful way to think about being trans?

Many trans philosophers have argued that it isn't. Julia Serano thinks that there's something troubling about starting from questions about why trans people transition. For one, these assumptions imply that transgender people are in need of explanation in a way that cisgender people aren't and hence that cisgender life is more 'natural' and not questionable.[13] Why, for instance, haven't we spent this chapter thinking about why cisgender people mostly fail to have the desire to transition? Writing in the volume *Transgender Marxism*, Xandra Metcalfe suggests that a focus on why trans people want to transition speaks to an underlying view of trans people as "an aberration from the cissexual subject, a swerve from an otherwise straight line".[14] The sort of view being criticised here treats being cisgender as normal and preferable to being transgender and assumes that trans people lack something or are disordered when compared with cis people. You might think that this set of assumptions is beginning our inquiry from the wrong place.

So, let's turn this inquiry on its head: why are there so many cis people? Why do so many people fail to question their gender and come out as trans? One potential answer might be something like the following: "*It's just natural* – people with penises naturally want to be men, and people without them naturally want to be women". However, this explanation runs into a number of problems, foremost amongst which is explaining why so much of our society is organised around policing the development of children to ensure that boys and girls grow up as distinct groups, shaming any male children who express femininity, and bullying female children who want to live out their lives as boys. If being cisgender were natural, you might think that such policing was unnecessary!

Perhaps instead the explanation for the huge numbers of cisgender people comes from this gendered policing. There's nothing natural about it – rather, children are made to repress any queer and trans feelings that might arise by the cisheterosexual social structures that they live under. The few that manage to hold onto such feelings will eventually come out as trans or queer, but the vast majority are shamed, bullied, and policed into becoming cisgender heterosexuals. Now, such a theory of the 'why' of being cisgender is far from complete. We would still need a story about where these social structures come from and why they're enforced. Metcalfe, for instance, explains the origins of this policing in psychoanalytic terms, arguing that it is the result of a quest for patriarchal domination.[15] Alternatively, an 'orthodox' Marxist might think that this sort of policing of the gender binary is a result of attempts to organise reproduction in ways that output a regular supply of workers.

However we go about developing this sort of theory, it looks like we have radically departed from a position that treats trans people as developmental aberrations or as fetishists. Instead of treating cisgender life as natural and inevitable, we begin to think of transgender life as something possible and perhaps even desirable.

TRANSFORMATIVE EXPERIENCE

Earlier in this chapter, we considered an explanation for transition in terms of rational calculation about social privilege and benefit. Whilst in the rest of this chapter I've suggested that there's something fishy about wanting a general explanation for transness, we might still think that there's an interesting question about rationality and transition: that is, is it ever *rational* for an individual to transition?

An answer to this question is going to rely on an account of what it is to be rational. Accounts of rationality vary a lot, but one way of spelling out what it is this: the rational person acts in ways that maximise their expected value. What does this mean?

Well, by way of example, suppose that you're offered one of two puddings – chocolate ice cream and salted caramel ice cream. Whilst you enjoy the taste of chocolate you *really really* enjoy the taste of salted caramel – so you'll get more enjoyment out of eating the latter than the former. If you're rational, then, you'll opt for the salted caramel ice cream for your pudding. This is the choice that will maximise your expected value.

Of course, in reality, things are often more complex than choosing between ice cream flavours. Some options will have drawbacks or costs that need to be considered in our decision-making, and sometimes we'll have to make a decision based only on probable outcomes, rather than certainties. Being rational might involve difficult deliberation in these cases! Regardless, the point, at least in this account of rationality, is to act so as to get the highest expected value given the chance of various outcomes and the drawbacks that might be present.

How does this play out in the case of gender transitions? We saw earlier that the cost-benefit analysis for transition generally looked bad if we only considered social privilege and oppression. Coming out as trans generally impacts one's social and economic status rather negatively. However, there are other factors to consider beyond things like one's likely pay rate and whether there is lots of medical research done on people like oneself. Think, for instance, of the sheer unhappiness and discomfort faced by so many trans people who suffer from dysphoria. For most, transition is the only way of alleviating such dysphoria. Even more pressing is the rate of suicide among trans people suffering from dysphoria. If one is suicidal due to dysphoria, then one appears to have extremely good reasons to transition. On a more positive note, we can look to the feelings of gender joy, the so-called 'gender euphoria' described by so many trans people as they transition, and the sense of community and love with other trans people. Such feelings seem like they pull in favour of transition.

So, is transition rational? Well, there certainly are drawbacks to transition – but there also look to be some real benefits. You might think that it's partly going to come down to exactly what someone values and how much they value it. Remember that in order to figure out whether choosing salted caramel ice cream was the rational choice, we had to specify that you valued the taste of salted caramel more than the taste of vanilla. So, if someone really values their current social status and position of relative privilege in a transphobic society and fears violence should they transition, perhaps they think that that's enough to outweigh distressing feelings of dysphoria and repressed anguish they feel towards the life that they might have led had they come out. Meanwhile, for many others, they may see the benefits of transition, especially the alleviation of dysphoria and the end of the feeling that they are living a lie, as outweighing potential discrimination they may face for being out as trans. Whether it is rational to transition will depend on the things you value and the context you find yourself in. Making a decision here may or may not be easy, but it will be possible in principle to say whether it was rational or not.

However, one might think that things aren't so simple. L.A. Paul has pointed out that sometimes we have *transformative experiences*.[16] These are experiences of something entirely new to us, that can teach us something that we couldn't have learned without experiencing it, or which personally transform us in ways that change who we are and reshape what we value.

Paul thinks that a key example of this sort of experience is having a child. Unless you actually go through the process of becoming a parent, you'll never know what it's like to have a child. Sure, there might be similar experiences (like getting a pet, for instance), but having a child is really just a different kind of thing, which you can't properly understand until you go through the process yourself. What's more, Paul thinks that in many cases, parents are deeply changed by the experience of having a child. They are transformed by this experience, such that what they care about and what they value are radically reshaped. Suppose that before you had a kid, you might have really valued time with your friends and your skydiving hobby. However, after having a child and becoming a parent, you aren't as keen to spend time with your friends: you could be spending that time doting on your child or having a brief moment alone to rest following another late night of interrupted sleep looking after your newborn. Meanwhile you just can't see the value of skydiving anymore. Becoming a parent has left you feeling a deep sense of responsibility towards your child, and you can't bear the thought of abandoning your child if something went wrong with your parachute.

Becoming a parent, along with other transformative experiences, poses difficult problems for rational decision making. Remember that in our account of rational action, we held fixed what we valued, and acted so as to maximise our expected results given those values. But now we have a type of experience which, when we choose to go through with it, radically changes who we are and what we value. How on earth could we make a rational choice if we don't have a fixed set of values against which to judge which action is best? At first glance, it seems difficult to see how we could ever rationally decide whether or not to undertake a transformative experience.

This might be a complication if one thinks, as Veronica Ivy does, that gender transitions are transformative experiences:

> For someone who transitions from, for example, a relatively stereotypical masculine male identity to a relatively stereotypical feminine female identity, nearly everything about her experiences will change. Moving through the world where people attribute a male gender is very different from moving through the world where people attribute a female gender, particularly in sexist, patriarchal societies such as ours. Men are typically afforded more space than women; women are more likely to be ignored in conversation; people are more comfortable being touched (casually on the arm during conversation, for example) by women; and so on. The way one relates with social and legal institutions is changed, particularly if the person has to navigate the often complicated systems of changing their sex/gender marker on identification such as a driver's license, birth certificate, or social security number. It may change one's tastes in clothing, or at least one's ability to express and participate in various clothing and gender presentation preferences. And in almost all cases, one's post-transition preferences will have shifted over time: it's impossible to predict what gender presentation preferences one will have post transition, and how those choices will feel like, and how they will affect others' interactions with oneself.[17]

This seems very plausible: transitioning can involve massive changes to what it is like to be you, and can have very big impacts on the sorts of thing you value and how much you value them.

For a somewhat sillier example than those Ivy raises, we might look at how many trans women start craving salty foods, especially pickles, after beginning a hormonal transition. For the person who hated pickles before transitioning, eating pickles might seem like an awful idea. However, the person they become after having transitioned gets a lot out of eating pickles.

Does this mean that it is impossible to make a rational decision about whether to transition or not? Ivy suggests that there are features of gender transitions that make them different from many other transformative experiences, and hence rational in certain cases. She begins by simplifying the outcomes of a decision of whether or not to transition into two camps: whether or not you will be happy afterwards. Hence there are four possible results of a transition decision: transition-happy, transition-unhappy, don't-transition-happy, and don't-transition-unhappy. Now, if gender transitions are transformative experiences, we don't know for certain whether you'll be happy or unhappy if you opt for a transition! However, as Ivy points out, we know that a trans person deciding not to transition overwhelmingly leaves them in the don't-transition-unhappy camp. Indeed, for many trans people, this boils down to a choice between suicide and gender transition.

Given that the likelihood of ending up don't-transition-happy is virtually zero for so many trans people, Ivy suggests that opting to transition is rational, because it is what professional gamblers call a 'freeroll'. A freeroll is a bet where the person placing the bet will be no worse off if they lose and will gain something if they win. According to Ivy's analysis, a trans person not transitioning virtually always leads to unhappiness or suicide, so the trans person has nothing to lose by throwing the dice on transitioning. They might still end up unhappy, but they were going to be unhappy (or worse) anyway! Moreover, they might end up in the transition-happy camp – and as such the decision to transition is rational.[18]

Is this analysis right? A lot is going to turn on whether we think Ivy's simplifying assumptions are right here. Perhaps the particular kinds of happiness and unhappiness that one can experience depending on whether or not one transitions should affect our decision-making process. Maybe happiness isn't even the right thing to be judging our outcomes by. There's also questions about how one can be sure that one is trans and hence subject to the kinds of predictions about life without transitioning that Ivy points out. Finally, we might think that whilst this analysis is right regarding the rationality of transition for suicidal closeted trans people, it leaves out a class of trans people for whom transition isn't life or death but rather a choice over whether to leave an uncomfortable but manageable life in the closet. Here, the choice is not a freeroll, and trying to make a rational case for transitioning (or indeed not transitioning) may be more difficult.

Of course, not every decision that we make needs to be justified on rational grounds. One of the important things that we can take away from Paul's work is that our lives are full of important decisions that can't always be made rationally. Transformative experiences reshape who we are and how we experience the world, often representing big moments of choice in our lives. It is perhaps appropriate then, that we can't just do a rational calculation to figure out what course of action to take. Instead, you might think, sometimes we need to just make a decision and stand by it, not relying on rationality to tell us the right thing to do. Sometimes, as the Danish philosopher Søren Kierkegaard argued, what is required for us to become the fully flourishing people we might one day be is a leap of faith into the unknown: whether a leap into parenthood or a leap into a gender transition.[19]

NOTES

1 Some of this work is being attempted. See e.g., Flint, C., Förster, K., Koser, S.A. et al. (2020). "Biological Sex Classification with Structural MRI Data Shows Increased Misclassification in Transgender Women". *Neuropsychopharmacology* 45: 1758–1765.

2 Gregory, Andrew. (2025). "'Concerning' Lack of Female-Only Medical Trials in UK, Say Health Experts". *theguardian.com*. https://www.theguardian.com/society/2025/may/07/concerning-lack-of-female-only-medical-trials-in-uk-say-health-experts (accessed 23 December 2025).

3 C.f., Raymond, Janice. (1994). *The Transsexual Empire: The Making of the She-Male*. New York and London: Teachers Press.

4 Overall, Christine. (2009). "Sex/Gender Transitions and Life Changing Aspirations", in Laurie Schrage (ed.) *"You've Changed": Sex Reassignment and Personal Identity*. Oxford: Oxford University Press, p. 14.

5 Cousens, Emily. (2023). *Trans Feminist Epistemologies in the US Second Wave*. New York and London: Palgrave Macmillan.
6 Blanchard, R. (1989). "The Concept of Autogynephilia and the Typology of Male Gender Dysphoria". *The Journal of Nervous and Mental Disease* 177(10): 616–623.
7 Serano, Julia. (2010). "The Case Against Autogynephilia". *International Journal of Transgenderism* 12(3): 179.
8 Serano, "The Case Against Autogynephilia", 181–182.
9 Bettcher, Talia Mae. (2007). "Evil Deceivers and Make Believers: On Transphobic Violence and the Politics of Illusion". *Hypatia* 22(3): 43–65.
10 C.f., Bettcher, Talia Mae. (2019). "What Is Trans Philosophy?". *Hypatia* 34(4): 644–667.
11 Pearce, Ruth. (2018). *Understanding Trans Health: Discourse, Power and* Possibility. Bristol and Chicago: Polity, p. 88.
12 Overall, "Sex/Gender Transitions", 23.
13 Serano, Julia. (2016). *Whipping Girl: A Transsexual Woman on Sexism and the Scapegoating of Femininity*. California: Seal Press.
14 Metcalfe, Xandra. (2021). "'Why Are We Like This?' The Primacy of Transsexuality", in Jules Joanne Gleeson and Elle O'Rourke (eds.) *Transgender Marxism*. London: Pluto Press, p. 219.
15 Metcalfe, "Why Are We Like This?", 223.
16 Paul, L.A. (2014). *Transformative Experience*. Oxford: Oxford University Press.
17 Ivy, Veronica (authored as Rachel McKinnon). (2015). "Trans*formative Experiences". *Res Philosophica* 92(2): 422.
18 Ivy, "Trans*formative Experiences", 423–425.
19 Kierkegaard, Søren. (2009). *Concluding Unscientific Manuscript*. Cambridge: Cambridge University Press.

RECOMMENDATIONS FOR FURTHER READING

In addition to the works already cited in this chapter, those wanting to think more about desire and transformative experience in the context of transgender philosophy might like to take a look at the following:

There is a *lot* of discussion about biology, nature, gender, and sexuality in the feminist literature. Key places to start thinking about these topics, along with 'born this way' narratives here include Simone de Beauvoir's classic *The Second Sex*:

Beauvoir, Simone de. (1949/2011). *The Second Sex*, Constance Borde and Seila Malovany-Chevallier (trans.). London: Vintage Books.

What might a theory of transition that sidesteps 'why' questions look like? Jules Joanne Gleeson instead presses us to think about the how of transition: taking it for granted that people want to transition, how do they go about transitioning?

Gleeson, Jules Joanne. (2021). "How Do Gender Transitions Happen?", in Jules Joanne Gleeson and Elle O'Rourke (eds.) *Transgender Marxism*. London: Pluto Press, pp. 70–84.

Questions around the desire for transition are taken up in E.M. Hernandez's remarkable chapter "Fuel to my Fire/You Can't Stop Desire". Drawing on sources as diverse as Iris Murdoch, John McDowell, Judith Butler, and Bernard Williams, Hernandez engages with questions surrounding the barriers to desiring transition and the demand for an explanation:

Hernandez, E.M. (Forthcoming). "Fuel to My Fire/You Can't Stop Desire", in Matthew Cull, Alexis Davin and Katharine Jenkins (eds.) *Trans Philosophy in a Time of Crisis*. London and New York: Bloomsbury.

In the same volume, I have a chapter that goes deeper on questions surrounding how and if it is possible to shape desire, especially the desires that others may have for our genders, and how we can disappoint them. It also looks at narratives surrounding the changeling, a creature of European folklore!

Cull, Matthew J. (Forthcoming). "Children as Commodity and Changeling: Gender Disappointments and Gender Disappointment", in Matthew Cull, Alexis Davin and Katharine Jenkins (eds.) *Trans Philosophy in a Time of Crisis*. London and New York: Bloomsbury.

Trans philosopher R.A. Briggs has an excellent *Stanford Encyclopedia of Philosophy* article on rationality as expected value:

Briggs, R.A. (2023). "Normative Theories of Rational Choice: Expected Utility". *Stanford Encyclopedia of Philosophy*. https://plato.stanford.edu/entries/rationality-normative-utility/

Transformative experiences have seen much discussion over recent years, with plenty of attempts to understand how they interact with rationality. Rebecca Chan's *Stanford Encyclopedia* article is a good place to start on this literature:

Chan, Rebecca. (2023). "Transformative Experience". *Stanford Encyclopedia of Philosophy*. https://plato.stanford.edu/entries/transformative-experience

5

COLONIALISM, RACE, AND THE HISTORY OF GENDER

Whilst much work in trans philosophy looks at gender as it is now, some of the most exciting developments in the field have come from thinking about the history of gender and how that history continues to impact the present. In this chapter we'll focus in particular on the history of gender as it relates to colonialism and the racialised chattel slavery that saw millions kidnapped from Africa and put to work in the 'New World'. As we'll see, there's good reason to focus on these histories in particular: several trans philosophers have argued that if we are to understand gender at all, we need to understand its role in colonial expansion and chattel slavery.

LUGONES AND THE COLONIALITY OF GENDER

There is no getting away from the fact that the history of European colonialism is tied up with gender and sexuality. As European nations expanded across the globe in the latter half of the last millennium, they took with them their overwhelmingly binary understandings of the 'proper' roles of men and women. Of course, European colonialism was intensely violent and repressive across the board, but Europeans seemed to take particular exception

DOI: 10.4324/9781003502944-6

whenever they came across people who seemed to violate their assumptions about gender and sexuality. Take, for instance, the following example of Spanish colonial conquest in Central America, where a conquistador had forty people torn apart by dogs:

> In a 1513 quest for the South Sea, the iron-clad army of Spanish commander Vasco Nuñez de Balboa traversed the Isthmus of Panama and into the tangled forest of Quarequa. After slaying over six hundred Cueva warriors 'like brute beasts', Balboa and his soldiers advanced towards the fallen cacique's palace in pursuit of gold, pearls and prisoners. What they discovered, however, was much more exotic than expected: forty 'young men in women's apparel, smooth & effeminately decked' in white cotton *naguas* (skirts), engaging in the 'preposterous venus' of sex. Rather than execute these 'filthy kind of men' on the spot, Balboa demanded they be dragged to the village centre and offered as prey to his mastiffs as spectacle.[1]

Making sense of this violence against indigenous persons who did not fit into the narrow categories of straight and cisgender has importance beyond just our understanding of history. In many places, indigenous resistance to the imposition of a binary gender system continues to this day. Consider, for instance, the open letter sent by the women of the Zapatista movement:

> they only speak of the equity of women and men, and even we, who they call ignorant and backward, we know well that there are people who are neither men nor women, who we call "otroas", but who can call themselves as they please, and it has not been easy for them to gain that right to be who they are without hiding, because they are mocked, persecuted, violated, murdered. Are we still going to force them to be either men or women?[2]

The Zapatista movement is a (mostly) indigenous resistance movement against the Mexican state and capitalist imperialism, and in the previous quote we see them rail against those who would impose manhood or womanhood on those with the indigenous gender otroa.

How then, should we make sense of colonialism and its relationship to gender? Many trans philosophers have here turned to the work of María Lugones. The Argentine feminist Lugones has become one of the central references in contemporary trans philosophy, with many philosophers drawing on her work to think about pluralism and how we navigate moves between different social contexts.[3] However, perhaps the area of trans philosophy that Lugones has had the most influence on is the study of the relationship between colonialism, gender, and transness. For Lugones, understanding the history of European colonial expansion is central to understanding gender.

At different points in her career, Lugones seems to say different things about what the exact relationship between colonialism and gender is. As Perry Zurn points out,

> Lugones developed her account of the "modern/colonial gender system", according to which *gender* refers to a sexual dimorphism that is expressed via white bourgeois categories of man and woman. In its first iteration, Lugones' locution leaves it unclear if gender predated (post-Medieval) European colonialism (e.g., she refers to Indigenous "third genders") or if gender itself originated with (post-Medieval) European colonialism. In its later iterations, Lugones is quite clear that gender – by which she means the atomic, homogenous, separable categories "man" and "woman" which obey categorial, dichotomous, and hierarchical logic – belongs to and originates with (post-Medieval) European colonial power.[4]

As such, there are two different accounts of the relationship between European colonialism and gender that we can draw from Lugones's work. First, an earlier, more moderate account that suggests that indigenous persons had genders prior to colonisation, but that these were not (always) the rigid binary genders that predominated in Europe at the time. Colonisation by Europeans involved a strict policing of gender, such that only a binary gender hierarchy and a straight sexuality were permitted. Second, a later, more radical account that suggests that indigenous persons did not have genders *at all* prior to colonisation. Colonisation by Europeans 'gave' indigenous peoples genders, violently imposing a gender hierarchy and sexuality that simply did not exist beforehand.

This latter, more radical view might sound surprising to you. Did indigenous people really not have gender prior to colonisation? Were there really no indigenous men and women until the Europeans showed up and imposed their gender system? Lugones's argument for this claim involves thinking about the worldview or ideology of the European colonisers. According to Lugones, "Indigenous peoples of the Americas and enslaved Africans were classified as not human in species – as animals, uncontrollably sexual and wild".[5] So, in the worldview of the colonisers, the indigenous and the enslaved were akin to animals. Animals might have a sex, but they don't have genders. Gender is a feature of human social life! Part of the so-called 'civilising mission' of colonists is to bring to the 'natives' human society, including gender.

The radical view isn't just an interesting claim about the history of gender. Lugones also thinks it has upshots for how we might build a better world today. Many feminists think of themselves as primarily concerned with fighting for women's rights or women's liberation. However, suppose that the radical version of Lugones's story is correct. Given that for colonised peoples, gender is a result of violent control and rule by European powers, it's unclear that we should be particularly attached to genders, whether *woman* or otherwise. As she writes, the feminist who is conscious of this history of colonialism should, "drop her enchantment with 'woman', the universal, and [begin] to learn about other resisters at the colonial difference".[6] Instead of being concerned with the rights of women, says Lugones, we ought to look to a variety of indigenous and person of colour communities to form a coalition.

Now, there are lots of things to say about this. For instance, we'll return to questions about going without gender in the next chapter. For now, instead let's think about issues facing Lugones's radical reading of colonial history as giving gender to the colonised. One issue for the radical account is that we take it that gender is *now* a worldwide phenomenon, but it's not as if every single society around the world was colonised by a European power. Take, for instance, Korea, which was only colonised starting in 1910, and not by a European power – rather, it was colonised by Japan. If gender is a European social structure imposed through colonialism, then it looks like Korean people don't have genders in Lugones's account.[7]

However, Lugones has a response available to her in responding to this objection: she can say that colonial power can and indeed has taken different forms across time. Sure, European powers in Africa and the Americas imposed colonial control through violence and direct government, but there are other ways for a powerful state to shape the society of another nation. They might attempt to exert economic control by blockading all the ports and imposing tariffs on trade with that nation. Or they might attempt to exert so-called 'soft power' through the export of their cultural products to the other nation. American denim, for instance, often became a symbol of rebellion in the Soviet Bloc, with jeans playing no small part in the youth culture that eventually led to the fall of the Berlin wall and the end of the Cold War. Whilst these alternative forms of colonial power tend to be characteristic of 20th and 21st century 'neocolonialism', rather than the colonialism of the era that Lugones is focused on, cultural exchange and economic power have always existed. Perhaps, then, Lugones might claim that gender was imposed on the Korean peninsula through cultural exchange with the European powers and the societies that the Europeans *had* in fact colonised.

With that said, I'm still sceptical that gender *originates* with European colonialism. There were plenty of practices in a variety of precolonial societies that looked a lot like gender as we know it today. Though not universal, there certainly were plenty of societies where labour and social roles were divided up according to the individual's (perceived) reproductive bodily features. There were also plenty of other kinds of social roles that looked (and indeed still look like) genders beyond the binary in indigenous society, including *fa'afāfine* and *hijra* – something we'll discuss more in the next section. Moreover, you might think that Lugones herself attributes too much authority to European conceptions of gender. Sure, Europeans of the time may have thought of indigenous and enslaved individuals as not persons and hence not having genders, and certainly in many cases they treated such individuals as not fully persons. However, why think that European colonial society of the time was the arbiter of who counts as having a gender prior to colonisation? Surely we can say that the coloniser's worldview is *just wrong*, or at least partial. Recalling Chapter 1, for instance, the pluralist about the metaphysics of gender might say that a fa'afāfine person does not have a gender according to colonial European conceptions of gender, but that they do have a gender (fa'afāfine) according to Samoan conceptions of gender.

Perhaps however, there is a way of holding onto some of Lugones's central insights about the influence European colonialism has had on gender without saying that European colonialism gave us gender entirely. This would likely involve endorsing her earlier, more moderate view: even if gender existed prior to colonisation, colonisation imposed a strict way of doing gender. If there wasn't a binary organised around perceived reproductive capacities before European colonisation, there definitely was afterwards!

What's nice about this more moderate position is that it helps us make sense of cases like that of Balboa setting his dogs on the people of Quarequa. According to the moderate reading, the indigenous peoples of Quarequa had gender. However, they seemed not have a strict gender binary and didn't have a prohibition on same-sex relationships in the same way as the Spanish did at the time. So, what occurred in this case is that Balboa and the other Spanish colonists violently imposed a strict heterosexual gender binary upon the indigenous people, killing those with genders and sexualities that were at odds with the Spanish way of thinking about gender.

Lugones's earlier position also helps us to make sense of the internal logic of many colonial enterprises. Consider, for instance, the self-professed goals of the Canadian residential school system. The residential school system was a longstanding institution developed by the Canadian government in conjunction with the Christian church that attempted to 'civilise' indigenous children by isolating them from their families and culture, instead attempting to raise such children in a Euro-Canadian culture. Of course, such a goal is deeply morally troubling, amounting to a form of cultural genocide according to a truth and reconciliation report.[8] The schools were sites of physical and sexual abuse, and unmarked graves continue to be found at a number of the schools. The last residential school only closed in 1997.

At the heart of the justification for the residential system was the belief that, in Captain Henry Pratt's words, they could "Kill the Indian in him, and save the man".[9] This line is hard to make sense of if we opt for Lugones's later, more radical reading. Certainly, Pratt and the other settlers thought of indigenous people as featuring an aspect that needed to be eradicated – their indigenous culture. However, contrary to the later Lugones's reading of colonial ideology, Pratt clearly thought that Indians have something akin to personhood and perhaps even gender that can be saved through appropriate enculturation. Lugones's earlier more moderate position gives us an easy interpretation of events: the colonists imposed their way of doing gender on the indigenous population of Canada through the residential school system. The indigenous peoples already had other forms of life, including ways of organising gender, before that. So, the colonists thus saw their task as one of stamping out these indigenous gender practices and replacing them with a strict gender binary.

TRANSGENDER NEOCOLONIALISM

Regardless as to whether one thinks the earlier or the later Lugones is right about whether indigenous peoples had gender prior to colonisation, both versions of Lugones agree that a strict binary and heterosexual gender system was imposed in European colonisation. European ways of thinking about gender were exported and used to organise the lives of people outside Europe. As mentioned previously, colonisation in the 20th and 21st centuries has taken on a variety of different, often more subtle forms in *neo*colonialism. In addition to traditional forms of colonialism, the more powerful nations today exert their power over other societies through things like cultural influence, economic strong-arming, and the global dominance of certain languages – especially English.

If colonialism isn't over but instead has continued, one might worry that certain forms of gendered life continue to be imposed in various forms of neocolonialism. One of the most interesting versions of this claim comes from indigenous philosophers who claim that, in addition to imposing *man* and *woman* as genders, European and especially North American neocolonialism imposes the gender category *transgender* on indigenous people.

One way of making this argument is to suggest that *transgender* is not a completely universal category but rather a historically and culturally specific one that emerges from a particular context: North American and European biomedical science in the 20th century. In this sort of story, the category usually begins with the pioneering work of Magnus Hirschfield's *Institute für Sexualwissenshaft* [Institute for Sexual Science] in pre-Nazi Berlin and develops in the United States at Johns Hopkins University's Gender Identity Clinic under the auspices of John Money. These were medical institutions, attempting to diagnose and treat people using the frameworks of European and American psychology and medicine. As such, the way of thinking about the category of *transgender* that developed in these institutions was one that had a number of idiosyncratic features characteristic of thinking about gender variance in terms of a psychiatric disorder – not least that it is something that is in need of treatment. One feature of much of this particular way of thinking about the category of *transgender* is that it assumes a gender binary and that individuals must seek to live 'convincingly' as either men or women.

Now, think of contexts where European and North American medical science is something that is imposed from outside and is perhaps even taken up enthusiastically by local medical professionals. You might think that those working in this tradition are going to use its particular way of understanding the category of *transgender* in order to categorise and interact with people whose genders are not straightforwardly cisgender men or women. So, whatever rich and varied gender variance existed before, variance that had only just been able to escape the imposition of a rigid gender binary in the original process of colonialism, now gets jammed into the new neocolonial categories of trans man and trans woman.

One thinker who offers a version of this argument is the travesti communist Lohana Berkins. Berkins points to two distinct ways in which narrow conceptions of gender are imposed upon travesti people. The first is imposed by the specific combination of economic poverty and patriarchal desire that travestis face in Argentina. Travestis, notes Berkins, have often only been able to gain an income through sex work. As she puts it, "Prostitution continues to be the only option. . . . We could talk about choice if we were able to access ordinary jobs".[10] Travestis thus faced an economic demand: become desirable to men, fulfilling their erotic fantasies, or else starve. Simonetto and Vidal-Ortiz put it like this:

> One such fantasy is what Berkins called, as noted before, "the 'prostibular' body": the fantastic, voluptuous, and at times exaggerated view of cisgender women that heteronormative men projected onto *travestis*, and/or which many *travestis* sought to develop . . . in order to feel desirable, and to earn money.[11]

So, a restrictive and hypersexualised femininity is imposed on travestis by their economic position and the desires of men in a patriarchal society.

The other narrow conception of gender imposed on travestis, according to Berkins, is that imposed by dominant narratives around what it is to be transgender. Berkins insists that we should draw a sharp distinction between *trans* and *travesti* on a couple of grounds. First, she suggests that the conception of transness at work outside of Latin America is one that involves being beholden to a gender binary in ways that travestis reject:

> travestis live in different circumstances with respect to those of us who come across transgender people from other countries, who frequently turn to sex reassignment surgeries and have as an objective to reconfigure themselves into the binary logic of male and female. A large amount of Latin American travestis assert the option to occupy a space outside of the binary movement, and it's our objective to destabilize the categories of male and female.[12]

Second, she contrasts the notion of *transgender* as developed in North American academia with *travesti* – which, as she points out, "comes to us from medicine, and has been reappropriated, reworked, and fleshed out by travestis to call themselves by that word".[13] According to Berkins, the unique history of travesti people's engagement and struggle with a medical establishment differentiates *travesti* from the notion of *transgender* employed by that medical establishment. Just as the prostibular body attempts to corral and constrain travesti life to a narrow vision of femininity, so too the category of transgender as employed by Western medical establishment attempts to constrain travesti to a binary mode of life that they reject.

Now, there's much more detail that one could add to this argument, especially regarding the seemingly differing histories of trans people's and travesti people's relationships with medical science. However, one thing that you might say is that this sort of critique of medicalised ideas about the category of transgender needn't be made in terms of colonialism and anticolonialism. After all, there are plenty of trans people in Europe and America who would feel and have felt that this sort of medicalised conception of transness was an imposition that didn't reflect who they really were. Many in such contexts have argued against a narrow understanding of transness as just trans men and trans women who must seek to live 'convincingly' as men and women respectively. Nonbinary people, for instance, have long argued for a broader notion of what it is to be transgender. Indeed, pushback from trans people has led to some degree of change in medical and psychiatric ideas about trans people.

Can the anticolonial critique be pushed any further? Possibly! For instance, we might buy the likes of Berkins's argument that the medical establishment's ideas around being transgender are a colonial imposition but also wonder whether it also applies to other ways of thinking about transgender. Take, for instance, the rather minimal concept of transgender that we've been working with for most of this book: a person is transgender if and only if they don't identify as a member of the gender that matches the gender that they were assigned at birth. This is one way of spelling out perhaps the most widespread conception of what it is to be trans today. Crucially, nothing about it implies that trans people must (for example) seek to conform to any gender binary, nor that they need to seek out gender affirming surgery in order to count as trans. So, it looks like a lot of Berkins's worries about other conceptions of the category *transgender* just don't apply to this more minimal conception.

However, we might still be worried that the more minimal conception of what it is to be transgender still involves a form of neocolonialism. This more minimal way of thinking about the category *transgender* largely emerges from a few sources: certainly, the medical tradition that we discussed previously had a part in its development, but perhaps more important were the American and European trans people negotiating with and reacting against that medical tradition, alongside various sources in North American academia and activism. As such, this way of thinking about what it is to be transgender emerges from a particular context – culturally, economically, and militarily dominant nations. That is, it is a concept that comes from the colonial powers – albeit (in no small part) from marginalised people within those colonial powers, who were often struggling against the state. Moreover, this conception of what it is to be transgender purports to be universal. That is, its definition makes no reference to cultural specifics: anyone anywhere and at anytime can turn out to be transgender, just so long as they happen to not identify with the gender that matches the sex that they were assigned at birth.

Why think that these features are troubling? Well, you might think that there's something going awry if the person from Europe were to insist to the likes of Berkins that "you might insist that travestis are not transgender, but we in North America and Europe have come up with a definition of being transgender by which you are wrong". On the one hand, this seems to run against an intuition that we should have something like a right to self-determination over our gender – a right that we are denying to Berkins by insisting on this definition of "transgender". On the other, you might argue that there's something morally suspect about the people in the colonial powers being the ones with the power and authority to determine who and what counts for this or that category and then imposing that judgement on others.[14] You might think of this as a kind of 'conceptual colonialism' – a rather troubling charge, and one with far-reaching consequences beyond just gender, at least if arguments of this sort can be made successfully! For instance: are *any* universal concepts developed in the colonial powers redeemable?

SNORTON ON TRANSNESS AS BOUND UP WITH BLACKNESS

A quite different perspective on the history of gender and trans life comes from C. Riley Snorton, who argues for the centrality of chattel slavery in the development of sex and gender. Snorton's argument draws on a variety of historical and literary sources, but here we'll take a look at just two of his central examples: the use of slaves in the development of gynaecology and the cross-dressing practices of those trying to escape slavery in the United States.

One of the most important medical scientists in the history of gynaecology is J. Marion Sims, a physician who worked in the USA in the 19th century. Sims developed a treatment for vesco-vaginal fistulas, which are holes in the wall between the bladder and the vagina that can be caused in pregnancy. Crucial in this treatment was his development of a precursor to the speculum – a device that allows easy access to orifices like the vagina by holding them open. Sims's work was incredibly influential, and modern gynaecology is a subject that owes much of its origins to Sims. Indeed, until recently a statue of him still stood in New York, opposite the New York Academy of Medicine.

In 2017, the statue was sprayed with the word 'racist' in red paint and was placed into storage shortly thereafter. Why? Well, one reason is that much of his work, especially in the treatment of fistulas and his development of the speculum, came from experimentation on enslaved Black women, procured from various slaveowners across the American South. The cruelty of these experiments can hardly be overstated. One woman, who was known as Anarcha, went through 30 separate experimental operations by Sims in the attempt to suture her fistula. To add insult to injury, "After applying his fistula procedures . . . Sims sent all of the named and unnamed captives back to their enslavers".[15]

What does Snorton want us to learn from this history of the very beginnings of modern gynaecology? Well, one thing is certainly that contemporary scientific understandings of the vagina and other aspects of bodies that are sexed as female begins in the racist exploitation of Black women slaves. So, our understandings of sex are deeply connected to race, historically at least. However, at times Snorton wants to go further and suggest that sex is not even possible without race.

According to Snorton, Black slaves did not have sexed bodies, properly speaking. The practice of chattel slavery dehumanised and objectified slaves to the extent that they were merely fungible 'flesh'. Fungible things are things that are interchangeable, as exemplified in commodities like oil. If you draw a litre of oil from a well, and I draw another litre of oil from the same well, we can swap our bottles of oil without either of us losing out – oil is fungible. According to Snorton, Black slaves were similarly just fungible commodities: interchangeable flesh for use in things like agriculture and medical experimentation. Snorton goes on to suggest that because it is in Sims's medical experimentation that modern ideas about sex (and gender) are developed, flesh is therefore a precondition for sex. So, flesh, in the form of racialised chattel slaves, is needed in order for us to get sex.

Being creatures of fungible flesh did, however, provide many slaves with a certain kind of opportunity, according to Snorton. What sort of opportunity? Well, in not having a sex or a gender (at least according to the dominant White society that such slaves were in) slaves could use cross-dressing practices to disguise themselves in order to escape from slavery. Take, for instance, the case of Ellen and William Craft. Ellen Craft, whose light skin allowed her to disguise herself as a White man, posed as a White master of a Black slave – her husband. With this cover story, the Crafts escaped their enslavement in Georgia to eventually arrive in the United Kingdom, where they would take part in the abolitionist movement. That Ellen's gender was fungible in the eyes of the White slaveholders allowed her to take on the guise of a man and escape, suggests Snorton.

Moreover, argues Snorton, "the inhabitation of the un-gender-specific and fungible also mapped the affective grounds for imagining other qualities of life and being for those marked by and for captivity".[16] One way to get a handle on what Snorton means here is that cross-dressing, for Snorton, is not just practical a way of escaping the plantation's slave-hunter. It is also a way of inventing new forms of life beyond the plantation. One might, for instance, draw a connection between the gender fungibility of Black slaves in the United States in the 19th century and the queer ballroom culture of African Americans in the 20th century, where expansive and beautiful modes of gendered life beyond a narrow gender binary were explored and lived.

One question we might put to Snorton is this: enslaved people were certainly treated as property, but in what sense were they really just fungible, unsexed flesh? It appears that many slaveowners were often very keenly aware of the sexed features of their slaves and employed this awareness in some of the cruellest ways imaginable. The history of male slaveowners raping and impregnating their female slaves, for instance, seems to suggest that slaveowners did not view all slaves as mere fungible flesh. Some had particular sorts of bodies that slaveowners sought to exploit. Moreover, recent historical scholarship has emphasised the way that slaveowners forced particular slaves to breed, often with the aim of improving their 'stock'. Former slaves in particular have emphasised this:

> For example, Charlotte Martin recalled that in Florida, her enslaver, Wilkinson, "found it very profitable to raise and sell slaves", and "selected the strongest and best male and female slaves and mated them exclusively for breeding". According to one [anonymous formerly enslaved person], enslavers in Kentucky only allowed "the strong healthy slave women . . . to have children", and often prevented them from "mat[ing] with their own husbands". Instead, their enslavers "bred them like live stock to some male. . . . who was kept for that purpose because of his strong physique". The respondent compared this selection process to livestock, stating that it was "just like [how] horses, cattle, dogs and other animals are managed today in order to improve the stock".[17]

So, many slaveowners seemed to be very keen to differentiate between different slave bodies, often in ways that involved sex, in part because they thought that they could breed 'better' slaves to put to work. This puts pressure on the sort of history of sex and gender that Snorton gives us: it looks like a (certain) understanding of sex was a necessary precondition for much of the practice of chattel slavery, and not the other way around!

You might also think it puts pressure on Snorton's account of fugitive genders. We might ask Snorton, for instance, why *cross-dressing* disguises were seen as useful by escaping slaves. If such enslaved people were ungendered and unsexed fungible flesh, surely it would have been enough for them to adopt *any* sort of gendered performance in their escapes! Yet the likes of Ellen Craft, a woman, seemed to see cross-dressing *as a man* as a vital part of her escape.

Regardless of whether this criticism of Snorton is correct, he is surely right to emphasise the role of racial slavery in the development of modern gynaecology and surgery. Even if we don't buy all of the historical claims that he develops, we still need to reckon with the racist origins of scientific practices that (among other things) today enable trans people to access bodies that they feel more at home in. The history of gender, sex, race, transness, and colonialism live on today, and making sense of how each is intertwined is crucial for both trans philosophy and making a better world tomorrow.

NOTES

1 Jesperson, Jamey. (2024). "Trans Misogyny in the Colonial Archive: Re-membering Trans Feminine Life and Death in New Spain, 1604–1821". *Gender & History* 36: 91–111.
2 Zapatista Women. (2019). "Letter from Zapatistas to Women Who Fight All Over the World", Abolition Media Worldwide (trans.). *InternationalViewpoint.org* https://internationalviewpoint.org/spip.php?article5944 (accessed 19 December 2025).
3 See, e.g., Bettcher, Talia Mae. (2025). *Beyond Personhood: An Essay in Trans Philosophy*. Minneapolis: University of Minnesota Press.
4 Zurn, Perry. (2024). "Trans Philosophy", in *Stanford Encyclopedia of Philosophy*. < https://plato.stanford.edu/entries/trans/ (accessed 18 December 2025).
5 Lugones, María. (2010). "Toward a Decolonial Feminism". *Hypatia* 25(4): 743.
6 Lugones, "Toward a Decolonial Feminism", 753.
7 I owe this point to Yuxuan Zhang and Jade Fletcher.
8 The Truth and Reconciliation Commission of Canada. (2015). "Honouring the Truth, Reconciling for the Future Summary of the Final Report of the Truth and Reconciliation Commission of Canada".

Publications of the Government of Canada. https://publications.gc.ca/collections/collection_2015/trc/IR4-7-2015-eng.pdf (accessed 19 December 2025).

9 Pratt, Richard Henry. (1892). "The Advantages of Mingling Indians with Whites", in Isabel C. Barrows (ed.) *The Proceedings of the National Conference of Charities and Correction*. Geo H. Ellis: Boston, p. 46.

10 Berkins, Lohana. (2019). *Selected Writings*, Jamie Berrout (trans.). River Furnace. https://www.patreon.com/posts/full-text-of-26491264, p. 10.

11 Simonetto, Patricio and Salvador, Vidal-Ortiz. (2025). "Lohana Berkins: A Latin American *Travesti* Theory of the Body". *Body and* Society 31(3): 11.

12 Berkins, *Selected Writings*, 22.

13 Berkins, *Selected Writings*.

14 C.f., many of the remarks in Binaohan, B. (2014). *Decolonizing Trans/Gender 101*. Toronto: Biyuti Publishing.

15 Snorton, C. Riley. (2017). *Black on Both Sides: A Racial History of Trans Identity*. Minneapolis: University of Minnesota Press.

16 Snorton, *Black on Both Sides*, 58–59.

17 Djelid, Aisha. (2024). "'The Master Whished to Reproduce': Slavery, Forced Intimacy, and Enslavers' Interference in Sexual Relationships in the Antebellum South, 1808–1861". *American Nineteenth Century History* 25(1): 23.

RECOMMENDATIONS FOR FURTHER READING

In addition to the works already cited in this chapter, some works that have been important philosophical contributions to the study of colonialism, race, and the history of gender include:

Scott Morgensen's work on queerness, settler colonialism, and indigeneity is an excellent place to look for those starting to think about these issues:

Morgensen, Scott Lauria. (2011). *Spaces Between Us*. Minneapolis: University of Minnesota Press.

Much work has been done linking contemporary transphobia to forms of settler colonialism. Drawing on Lugones, alongside a variety of other sources, Nishant Upadhyay gives us a nice short version of the argument:

Upadhyay, Nishant. (2021). "Coloniality of White Feminism and Its Transphobia: A Comment on Burt". *Feminist Criminology* 16(4): 539–544.

As mentioned, Lugones's influence on trans philosophy is extensive. For further examples of some of this influence that emphasise other aspects of her work than what we focused on in this chapter, see:

Bettcher, Talia Mae. (2014). "Trapped in the Wrong Theory: Rethinking Trans Oppression and Resistance". *Signs: Journal of Women in Culture and Society* 39(2): 383–406.

Hernandez, E.M. (2024). "Moral Shock and Trans 'Worlds' of Sense". *Journal of the American Philosophical Association* 10(4): 761–779.

Other travesti philosophers like PJ DiPietro and Giuseppe Campuzano are becoming increasingly influential in trans philosophy. In these texts, for instance, DiPietro develops the notion of 'sideways selves' an interesting and powerful tool, whilst Campuzano pulls together the history of gender in Peru with a call for liberatory politics:

Campuzano, Giuseppe. (2006). "Reclaiming Travesti Histories". *IDS Bulletin* 37(5): 34–39.

DiPietro, P.J. (2025). *Sideways Selves: Travesti and Jotería Struggles Across the Américas*. Texas: University of Texas Press.

Two key figures who have inspired much of Snorton's work are Hortense Spillers and Sylvia Wynter. Spiller's essay "Mama's Baby, Papa's Baby" has become a touchstone for many trans theorists of race and gender, whilst an excellent place to start with Wynter's work is her long essay "Unsettling the Coloniality of Being/Power/Truth/Freedom":

Spillers, Hortense. (1987). "Mama's Baby, Papa's Maybe: An American Grammar Book". *Diacritics* 17(2): 65–81.

Wynter, Sylvia. (2003). "Unsettling the Coloniality of Being/Power/Truth/Freedom: Towards the Human, After Man, Its Overrepresentation – An Argument". *CR: The New Centennial Review* 3(3): 257–337.

There are a variety of attempts to investigate the history of gender variance beyond those we've discussed here. For a recent and interesting account of that history in Europe, see DeVun's excellent *The Shape of Sex*. One area of extensive scholarship is in the study of eunuchs in Byzantine society. A place to start is with some of the essays in James's *Women, Men, and Eunuchs: Gender in Byzantium*:

DeVun, Leah. (2021). *The Shape of Sex: Nonbinary Gender from Genesis to the Renaissance*. New York: Columbia University Press.

James, L. (ed.). (1997). *Women, Men, and Eunuchs: Gender in Byzantium*. Abingdon: Routledge.

6

GENDER ABOLITION

When something is oppressive, harming us, or just downright unpleasant, one obvious thought we might have is this: let's get rid of it. Suppose you and I have being buying one another more and more expensive gifts each year for one another's birthdays. This practice started off from a place of goodwill – we wanted to treat our friend to a nice gift – but now things have got out of hand. There's a gift-based arms race, with each of us spending more and money each year. It has become financially unsustainable. We should, you might think, stop our gifting practice. We can sit down together and *abolish* our birthday rituals. Of course, this example of abolition is small scale and perhaps a little silly. But there have been some hugely significant campaigns for the abolition of globe-spanning social practices, most famously the various fights for the abolition of slavery.

Now, gender isn't slavery, nor is it a birthday ritual. But it sure does look like the kind of thing that hurts and oppresses us. From transphobic violence to stereotypes about what little girls can grow up to be, gender seems to be a prime candidate for the sort of thing that we should get rid of. And yet, surely things can't be so simple. Whilst we certainly are subject to serious harms that

DOI: 10.4324/9781003502944-7

come from gender, many trans people are invested in being men, being women, being genderqueer, and so on. Getting rid of gender seems like it would do harm to such people, or at least remove a certain kind of joy they experience in being able to live as a man, woman, or genderqueer person. Trans philosophers have hence been keen to explore this tension, taking up a variety of positions on the central question of this chapter: Should we abolish gender?[1]

GENDER OPPRESSION

Trans philosophers tend to begin from the assumption that there is something deeply troubling about our gendered world. Examples of the kinds of injustice we tend to have in mind are endless, from gendered wage disparities and sexual violence to uneven distributions of labour and verbal harassment. In whatever way we look at our world it seems like trans people and cisgender women suffer from gendered forms of oppression and subordination. Even cisgender men look like they suffer in various ways from gendered roles, expectations, and violence.

Of course, this oppression is not uniform. The particular ways in which (say) the street harassment of woman occurs can vary wildly, not least due whether the victim is perceived to be cis or trans. What's more, this gendered oppression interacts with other forms of oppression, from racism and homophobia to ableism and xenophobia. These 'intersectional' oppressions vary hugely, and have sometimes been given their own names. For instance, Moya Bailey coined the term 'misogynoir' to refer to the specific blend of racism and misogyny that she and others face as Black women.[2]

It seems, then, that gender is bound up with an array of awful practices of oppression and violence. And, one might think, there's a fairly simple argument to be made here:

1. We should abolish anything that gives rise to oppression, violence, or subordination.
2. Gender gives rise to sexist and transphobic oppression, violence, and subordination.
3. Therefore: we should abolish gender.

We'll return to the question of whether we should buy this argument in a moment, but first let's think about how trans people might react to the idea that gender should be abolished. You might think that there are going to be lots of trans people who are awfully wary of the abolition of gender. After all, many trans people express their identity in terms of *wanting to be a man, living my authentic life as a woman,* or *feeling fulfilled in my genderqueer identity.* Such trans people seem to want to keep gender, not abolish it. After all, if you get rid of gender, and hence get rid of being a man, how is it possible for a trans man to fulfil their desire to be a man or live authentically as a man?

Trans philosophers, then, seem to be pulled in two different directions. On the one hand, the reality of transphobic gendered oppression lends itself to a call for the abolition of gender. On the other hand, many trans people's experiences of gender and desires for certain kinds of gendered life pull trans philosophers towards a position that opposes the abolition of gender.

MIKKOLA'S RESPONSE

One way to resolve this dilemma is to argue that the simple argument for the abolition of gender doesn't work. But where might this argument fail? Mari Mikkola gives us one way of trying to reject the simple argument:

> Abolitionist accounts take womanhood to be by definition tied to oppression so that it is not possible to be a woman and not be (in some sense) oppressed. Re-evaluative accounts do not take being a woman per se to be oppressive. Instead, they recognize that our social circumstances create environments where women are viewed and treated in ways that disadvantage them – perhaps by associating with women some traits and using this association to ground unjust social arrangements. It is possible to be a woman and yet not be oppressed, provided that we have successfully altered how women are viewed and treated. So, on the former view, gender justice would dismantle unjust social hierarchies, thus doing away with women and men; on the latter, gender justice would dismantle such hierarchies while retaining women and men without (say) the earlier oppressive association in place.[3]

The thought that Mikkola expresses is that even if gender *currently* gives rise to subordination or violence, that doesn't mean that it always will give rise to subordination or violence. Perhaps we can change things so that gender no longer gives rise to subordination or violence. So, the problem with the simple argument lies in that Premise 1 ("We should abolish anything that gives rise to oppression, violence, or subordination") is false. We have other options than abolishing gender: we might *change gender* such that it no longer gives rise to subordination, oppression, or violence. Perhaps things like gender as a hierarchical social structure do need to be eliminated, but we might hold onto gender as identity, gendered aesthetics, gender categories, and certain interpersonal gender roles, should it be possible to remove their contribution to gendered oppression.

GENDER NIHILISM

Some trans philosophers are unhappy with a Mikkola-style response to the simple argument, however, and argue that we should still abolish gender. Perhaps the most forceful statement of this kind of position comes from the gender nihilist tradition, exemplified in the work of Alyson Escalante:

> We are radicals who have had enough with attempts to salvage gender. We do not believe we can make it work for us. We look at the transmisogyny we have faced in our own lives, the gendered violence that our comrades, both trans and cis have faced, and we realize that the apparatus itself makes such violence inevitable. We have had enough. . . . All we demand in the present is a relentless attack on gender and the modes of social meaning and intelligibility it creates.[4]

Crucial to Escalante's argument here is the *inevitability* of violence. Escalante and other gender nihilists tend to regard the links between gender and things like oppression, subordination, and violence as *necessary* connections. That is, there is no change that we could make to gender that would stop it giving rise to oppression, subordination, and violence. Escalante argues that recent attempts to broaden gender beyond the man/woman binary won't end the deep and necessary connection between gender and oppression:

> All we do when we expand gender categories is to create new more nuanced channels through which power can operate. We do not liberate ourselves, we ensnare ourselves in countless and even more nuanced and powerful norms. Each one a new chain.
>
> To use this terminology is not hyperbolic; the violence of gender cannot be overestimated. Each trans woman murdered, each intersex infant coercively operated on, each queer kid thrown onto the streets is a victim of gender. The deviance from the norm is always punished. Even though gender has accounted for deviation, it still punishes it. Expansions of norms is an expansion of deviance; it is an expansion of ways we can fall outside a discursive ideal. Infinite gender identities create infinite new spaces of deviation which will be violently punished. Gender must punish deviance, thus gender must go.[5]

If Escalante and the other gender nihilists are correct about the necessary connection between gender and oppression, then there is an updated version of the simple argument for gender abolition that we can put forward:

1a. We should abolish anything that *necessarily* gives rise to oppression, violence, or subordination.
2a. Gender *necessarily* gives rise to sexist and transphobic oppression, violence, and subordination.
3a. Therefore: we should abolish gender.

A Mikkola-style response won't work here: we can't change gender in order to stop it giving rise to oppression, because it necessarily gives rise to oppression. Whenever there's gender, there's also oppression! According to this version of the argument, there is no way to have gender in a society without it giving rise to things like sexism and transphobia.

Is there a way to respond to the gender nihilist reformulation of the simple argument? Well, one way might be to draw on the sorts of distinctions that we made in Chapter 1, between different senses of the term 'gender'. You might say something like the following:

> Trans people who want to preserve gender are mostly interested in gender as identity. When they say 'I am a woman' they tend to mean it in the gender as identity sense and want to be able to live out their lives in line with that identity. Meanwhile gender abolitionists are mostly interested in the problems raised by gender as interpersonal interactions and gender as social structure, whether oppressive gender roles leading to violence or subordinating gendered social structures giving rise to uneven distributions of rights and income. So, the gender abolitionist and the gender preserver are just talking past one another: everyone can agree to preserve gender as identity and to abolish gender as social form.

Whilst a neat attempt to undermine the conflict, I'm not convinced by this response. Why? Well, for one, it's unclear what exactly gender as identity looks like in a world where gender as interpersonal treatment and social structure have been abolished. If there is no interpersonal or social significance to gender, it seems hard to see what one is identifying with when one identifies as this or that gender. Now, if we think that gender is mutable, then what one is identifying with might look very alien to contemporary gender roles and social structures, but gender as identity requires at least some interpersonal or social background in order to make sense at all.

In my previous work, I have attempted to provide a response to the gender nihilist's argument by denying 2a. That is, I don't think that it is possible to establish that gender *necessarily* gives rise to sexist and transphobic oppression:

> Whilst Escalante is correct to emphasise the violence experienced by those who deviate from gender norms, note that the world need not be this way. Let us grant for the moment that power is conceptually connected to gender and that power inevitably generates norms of behaviour. Even so, there's nothing to suggest that violent punishment necessarily follows from deviation from the norm. We can imagine a society

> where trans women are not murdered, intersex children are not coercively operated on, and queer children are not thrown out onto the streets. Indeed, is that not precisely what we ought to be fighting for?[6]

So, at least in my view, 2a is false. Sure, gender right now is embroiled in all sorts of discriminatory practices, oppression, violence, and so on. But it need not be this way. We can hold onto gender without, for instance, insisting that certain roles follow from a given gender identity. We can build a society where a doctor's exclamation of "It's a girl!" doesn't entail a constrained, oppressed, or second-class life. And a part of how this might be achieved is by looking at the kinds of resistance to gender oppression and subordination already underway in trans and feminist communities.

REASONS FOR KEEPING GENDER

Supposing that both the simple argument and its gender nihilist reformulation can be shown to be wrong, we might think that we've undermined (at least some of!) the reasons to be a gender abolitionist. But what about the positive case for *preserving* gender? In my recent work, I have attempted to give reasons for being a gender preserver.[7]

One reason that we gestured towards earlier was the thought that gender is very important to most trans people. Many *desire* to be a woman, *feel fulfilled* in living as a man, or say that they are *living authentically* in an androgyne identity. You might think that this is as good a reason as any to hold onto gender: it allows trans people to flourish, feel fulfilled, meet their desires, and live authentic lives. Meanwhile, when trans people are prevented from living gendered lives in the various ways that are fulfilling to them, we see that that trans people suffer horribly. Gender dysphoria, depression, suicidality, and a variety of other negative outcomes often arise when trans people aren't allowed to live their lives in the genders they identify with. So, you might think that retaining gender allows us to create a world in which trans people's suffering is reduced.

Will this convince the gender abolitionist? Perhaps not. To see why, we need to remember that most gender abolitionists see their political project as one that is going to involve a radical reshaping of society, one that will fundamentally reshape not just how we interact with one another but also how we see ourselves. So many gender abolitionists are interested in a society which has been changed so thoroughly by the abolition of gender that even trans people's experiences of themselves as gendered has been reshaped.

Take the example of gender dysphoria – the experiences of discomfort and distress at certain gendered aspects of one's body and social life felt by many trans people. What would this look like 'after the revolution', in a world where gender has been abolished? Well, the gender abolitionist might suggest that in their utopia there might be feelings of discomfort and distress at particular bodily features, but these could not be feelings of discomfort and distress at *gendered* bodily features, because there are no gendered bodily features in an abolitionist society! There are just bodily features, none of which are associated with gender at all. So, there is no such thing as gender dysphoria once we've abolished gender. Therefore, worries about people suffering gender dysphoria once gender has been abolished cannot be a good reason to preserve gender.

However, let's think through what this might look like. Take the case of two people: one, Sigrid, lives in our current society, and another, Emil, lives in a future hypothetical abolitionist society. Both Sigrid and Emil suffer from discomfort and distress at their penis, their facial hair, the distribution of fat on their body, their lack of breasts, and their lack of a vagina. Sigrid, in our current society, might see themselves as having gender dysphoria and hence seek out gender-affirming care to alleviate their suffering and aid them in leading a flourishing life as a transfemme genderqueer person. This gender-affirming care might take the form of feminising hormones and surgery to remove their penis and construct a vagina. What about the Emil in the hypothetical gender abolitionist society? Well, we might think that they see themselves as suffering from a kind of *body* dysphoria across a wide variety of body parts, and they might seek out treatment to alleviate their suffering, perhaps taking hormones to redistribute their body fat and having surgery to remove their penis and construct a vagina. Such treatment alleviates their symptoms of distress and discomfort and allows them to flourish in a gender-free world.

What should we make of this case? Well, on the one hand, the gender abolitionist can point to it and say, "Look, our society can care for people who in your society might count as trans! We can treat all of the same symptoms of distress and discomfort that you can, *and* we got rid of gender!" However, on the other, it seems like Sigrid in our current society has something that Emil in the genderless society does not have: a coherent story about the symptoms of distress and discomfort that she faces. This story provides a useful diagnostic tool, allowing both Sigrid and any medical professionals that might become involved to give a coherent account of why Sigrid is suffering from this particular set of bodily distresses and discomforts. It also provides Sigrid with a conceptual tool that allows her to make sense of her identity going forward: this wasn't a case of a random assortment of bodily distress and discomfort but rather her beginning to come to terms with the fact that she wasn't a man and was instead a transfemme genderqueer person.

One way to think about what is lacking for Emil in the hypothetical abolitionist society is that they are suffering from a hermeneutical injustice, as discussed in Chapter 3. In getting rid of gender, the abolitionist has removed an important set of tools that people had been using to make sense of their lives, their bodies, and their social worlds.

Now, this worry about hermeneutical injustice might leave the abolitionist unswayed. They might say that, in their utopia, there just is no need for a unifying diagnosis of Emil's various bodily discomforts and distresses. They might claim that this particular set of bodily symptoms will not arise with any regularity after the revolution, as it is only due to the existence of gender that we regularly see this pattern of symptoms, which is associated with transfeminine people and trans women. Emil wouldn't need to make sense of their symptoms as a coherent set of features: once the revolution has happened and gender has been abolished, gender concepts like a diagnosis of transfeminine gender dysphoria won't be useful in making sense of people's lives, bodies, and social worlds, as gender won't exist anymore. Indeed, there won't be many, or indeed any, Emils. However, I'm less convinced by this response from the gender abolitionist, largely because it relies on a speculative empirical claim about what sorts of dysphoric symptoms would tend to arise in their utopia.[8] We of course can't test this claim without going out and doing the gender abolitionist revolution!

WHAT LIES BENEATH: THREE OPTIONS

Let's set aside these arguments for a moment and assume that the abolitionist is right: we should get rid of gender! At this point we might ask, well, what's left? What does our society look like when we've excised gender? What do *we* look like once gender has been abolished?

An answer to the last of these questions may involve thinking about who we 'really' are, underneath all the gendered stuff that so dominates our lives right now. Once we've stripped away gender in the abolitionist future, you might think that we'll just be left without authentic selves. So, who are we, underneath all the gender? One answer to this question goes all the way back to the ancient Greek philosopher Plato. In his dialogue *The Symposium*, Plato has one of his characters, Aristophanes, tell a story about the nature of humanity and love:

> First you must learn what Human Nature was in the beginning and what has happened to it since, because long ago our nature was not what it is now, but very different. There were three kinds of human beings, that's my first point – not two as there are now, male and female. In addition to these, there was a third, a combination of those two; its name survives, though the kind itself has vanished. At that time, you see, the word "androgynous" really meant something: a form made up of male and female elements, though now there's nothing but the word, and that's used as an insult. My second point is that the shape of each human being was completely round, with back and sides in a circle; they had four hands each, as many legs as hands, and two faces, exactly alike on a rounded neck.[9]

Aristophanes continues at length, describing how humans were, in such a form, too powerful and threatened the gods. Zeus, king of the gods, thus came up with a cunning plan: he would split them in two. Each of us humans today is hence a broken remnant, seeking out our other half:

> Love is born into every human being; it calls back the halves of our original nature together; it tries to make one out of two and heal the wound of human nature.
>
> Each of us, then, is a "matching half" of a human whole, because each was sliced like a flatfish, two out of one, and each of us is always seeking the half that matches him.[10]

The male/female gender binary, along with love between couples, is, in Aristophanes' story, thus something that was made. Our true nature, which was ripped cruelly from us by the gods, involves us living as doubled creatures! Now, whilst this is a beautiful story that gives us both a supposed explanation for the origin of love and a radical reimagining of human nature, we should probably avoid taking Aristophanes' tale *too* literally. More than a few people have climbed Mount Olympus at this point, and there doesn't seem to be any sign of Zeus or any other god living up there after all! Moreover, its role in the broader dialogue is not as a straightforward recitation of what the author (Plato) thinks of underlying human nature – Aristophanes' speech is followed by other speakers whom Plato seems to accord greater esteem, not least Socrates. Plato's dialogue does, however, represent one beginning in a long history of people thinking about what our true nature might be, hidden away behind a constructed gender system, and what we might have lost by organising our lives around a gender binary.

Another approach to 'what lies beneath' the gendered world is to emphasise that the gendered world imposes on us tight restrictions and gives us only a narrow set of ways we might live. If you're assigned female at birth, you're likely going to spend the rest of your life being told that you need to love men, dress femininely, and otherwise *be a woman*. Even if you do end up identifying as a woman, enjoy dressing femininely, and find joy in a heterosexual partnership, you might worry that you only do those things because you've been told that's who you are and what you ought to do for your whole life. Gender, in this view, is an imposition. It's a set of restrictions on our freedom that prevent us from finding out who we really are and what we really want.

Think of, for instance, a young man who begins to feel a longing for the intimate company of other men, a desire to perform on stage, and jealousy at the beauty of the dresses his female friends wear when they attend events. In a freer society, we might think that he might begin to live life as a queer man and drag queen! But in a more repressive society, he might face intense backlash, public shaming, bullying from friends, and even legal retribution for attempting to live out these desires. So instead, he stays in the closet and represses those desires, pushing them down until he doesn't have to think about them anymore. You might think that he even begins to deny that those desires ever existed even to himself!

If we're so constrained by gender, you might think that our authentic selves, were they free from gender, would be radically different from how we currently appear to be. One influential idea about our underlying nature, drawing on the work of Sigmund Freud, is that we are 'polymorphously perverse' creatures. What does this mean? Well, in Freud's work on childhood development, he suggested that children were not free of sexual desire but rather expressed it in all sorts of ways and through all sorts of body parts that adults do not. Moreover, such children do not (yet) have fixed identities and senses of themselves as gendered. However, as we grow and are taught how to live in a gendered society, we form fixed identities and repress those desires that do not fit neatly with those identities.[11]

Many radical activists took up this idea in the 20th century. They argued that whilst we are (deep down) beings who have all sorts of desires and want to live in all sorts of different ways, dominant patriarchal society tells us that there are only men and women, that men must desire women, and that women must desire men. That society gives us a narrow set of categories that set out how we might live and asks us (whether through education, violent force, or just social pressure) to repress any desires or ideas that might suggest otherwise. In this sort of account, liberation and true freedom can only come from uncovering this underlying polymorphous perversity that is latent in all of us and throwing off the shackles of a society that forces us into cisgender and heterosexual boxes. Hence this position is gender abolitionist but also sexuality abolitionist: no more gender categories, and no more sexuality categories. Just polymorphously perverse individuals desiring one another and living truly freely.[12]

However, even supposing that this Freudian story is right about human infancy, it's unclear that there continues to be an underlying individual, which is deep down and hiding away in adulthood. Another story that drew on the same sorts of developmental biology might say that we start off as polymorphously perverse individuals, but then as we develop and are shaped by society, we become the sorts of creatures that have settled gender and sexual identities. Nothing is hidden away or repressed; there's no deep down 'real' polymorphous perversity inside each of us: we're just the sort of creatures that exist in and are shaped by the societies we live in. Moreover, perhaps the development of the human person requires some sort of socialisation and some set of categories with which to organise its life. Maybe those categories don't have to be as repressive and narrow as the ones we have now, but you might think that we need some sense of who we are and how we relate to one another in more systematic ways than just as genderless polymorphously perverse individuals.

You might also think that this is all a bit too *out there*. Sure, we might look a bit different once gender is abolished, but will we really be these radically different polymorphously perverse creatures? Another approach to thinking about what we'll look like once we do away with gender is by analogy to sci-fi societies which organise themselves into social hierarchies based on bodily features that we don't think are particularly significant.

> Imagine that we travelled to a far-off planet filled with humans whose society was divided into two 'gwaed' groups: the *aye*s and the *bae*s. The ayes are privileged in this society, whilst the baes face all sorts of discrimination. This gwaed social system is very old, and there are a variety of customs and cultures associated with ayes and baes, with ayes tending to dress and act very differently from baes. What determines whether someone is an aye or a bae? Well, every baby in this society is given a blood test at birth. Those with type-A blood are raised as ayes, and those with type-B blood are raised as baes. Of course, this social structure is not without its critics. There are bae-rights groups who call for better treatment of baes, and

> type-O blood activists who claim that they are neither ayes nor baes. There are even radical political groups who call for the overthrow of the gwaed system.

There's much that we might say about this society and its relationship to our own. But one thing to note is that our society is one that is free from a gwaed-based social structure. Those radicals in gwaed society might point to our society and say that we've abolished gwaed and we are what their society should look like. So what? Well, it suggests that one way of thinking about what we'll look like absent some powerful and all-encompassing social structure like gwaed or gender is that we'll be pretty boring. Not having gwaed in our society hasn't culturally impoverished us or left us as radically free individuals. So, the thought is, we won't uncover some polymorphously perverse authentic self – instead we'll just not organise our lives around the blood type or gender that we were assigned at birth. Gender abolition, in this sort of view, will be a pretty uninteresting change, at least in terms of what it does to us as individuals.

Of course, this analogy is not without its issues. You might think that there's something different between two relevant cases here: On the one hand, moving from a society which has some oppressive social system to one where is has been abolished, and on the other hand, being in a society that never had that oppressive system in the first place. It seems plausible to think that gender or gwaed *abolition* (as opposed to mere absence) would have huge impacts on our lives, perhaps upending who we think we are. But not having it in the first place will of course mean that its absence looks 'boring'! Moreover, one might argue that *of course* our gwaed-free society is boring and hasn't uncovered our polymorphously perverse selves: we've still got gender structuring our lives and desires! It is only once we free ourselves from *all* oppressive social structures that we'll finally be free to live in this authentic way.

Now, it's far from clear who wins out in this debate. Would a true abolition of gender leave us looking like Aristophanes' androgynous beings, as polymorphously perverse creatures, just boring genderless creatures for whom the abolition of gender will leave life looking pretty much the same as it always has, or something else entirely? Regardless, these various options do potentially provide the gender abolitionist with the beginnings of answers to a challenge that the abolitionist needs to respond to: what will we be like after gender? Moreover, will we like what we've become?

NOTES

1 The first half of this chapter draws on Cull, Matthew J. (2019). "Against Abolition". *Feminist Philosophy Quarterly* 5(3).
2 Bailey, Moya. (2021). *Misogynoir Transformed: Black Women's Digital Resistance*. United States: NYU Press.
3 Mikkola, Mari. (2016). *The Wrong of Injustice: Dehumanization and Its Role in Feminist Philosophy*. Oxford: Oxford University Press, p. 125.
4 Escalante, Alyson. (2016). "Gender Nihilism: An Anti-Manifesto". *libcom.org*.https://libcom.org/article/gender-nihilism-anti-manifesto-alyson-escalante
5 Escalante, "Gender Nihilism".
6 Cull, "Against Abolition".
7 Cull, Matthew J. (2024c). *What Gender Should Be*. London and New York: Bloomsbury, pp. 157–173.
8 Cull, *What Gender Should Be*, 163.
9 Plato. (1989). *Symposium*, Alexander Nehamas and Paul Woodruff (trans.). Indianapolis and Cambridge: Hackett, p. 25.
10 Plato, *Symposium*, 27.
11 See especially Freud's *Three Essays* in Freud, Sigmund. (1953). *The Standard Edition of the Complete Psychological Works of Sigmund Freud Volume VII*, James Strachey, Anna Freud, Alix Strachey and Alan Tyson (trans.). London: The Hogarth Press.
12 I discuss this radical tradition in Cull, *What Gender Should Be*, Chapter 7.

RECOMMENDATIONS FOR FURTHER READING

In addition to the works already cited in this chapter, those wanting to think more about abolition in the context of transgender philosophy might like to take a look at the following:

The idea of *intersectionality*, mentioned at the beginning of the chapter, has come to the forefront of feminist thought in recent years, in no small part due to the work of Kimberlé Crenshaw, who coined the term:

Crenshaw, Kimberlé. (2017). *On Intersectionality: Essential Writings*. New York: The New Press.

An early and radical from of transgender gender abolitionism comes from Martine Rothblatt, who ties the project of gender abolition to a form of transhumanism, transcending not just gender but the limitations of human biology entirely:

Rothblatt, Martine A. (1995). *The Apartheid of Sex: A Manifesto on the Freedom of Gender*. New York: Crown Publishing.

There are many trans philosophers who argue for a form of gender abolition via gender proliferation. The thought here is generally that once we have radically opened up our social practices to a huge variety of new genders, gender as a social form of control and subordination will wither away. See, for example:

Belinsky, Zoe. (2019). "Gender and Family Abolition as an Expansive and not Reductive Process". *medium.com*. https://medium.com/@malkekv-machashayfele/gender-and-family-abolition-as-an-expansive-and-not-reductive-process-d933f1f71da2 (accessed 24 October 2022).

Bjegunac, Stani. (2019). "Trans-cending the Market: How Socialist Planning Can Meet the Needs of Transgender People". *Cosmonaut Magazine*. https://cosmonautmag.com/2019/09/trans-cending-the-market-how-socialist-planning-can-meet-the-needs-of-transgender-people/ (accessed 24 October 2022).

Hester, Helen. (2018). *Xenofeminism*. Polity Press.

Daniel Weltman has recently argued for gender abolition, *but not yet*! For Weltman, the project of gender abolition is utopian, not an immediate practical recommendation. Pragmatically, we ought to hold off on gender abolition, even if it might be a worthwhile end goal.

Weltman, Daniel. (2024). "What Do We Want? To Eliminate Gender! When Do We Want It? Later!". *Pacific Philosophical Quarterly*, 105: 510–540.

The best contemporary interpretation of Aristophanes' speech in the *Symposium* comes as a part of a trans narrative in the cult film *Hedwig and the Angry Inch*:

Mitchell, John Cameron. (2001). *Hedwig and the Angry Inch*. New Line Cinema. (Film)

The radical 20th-century theorists taking up Freud's polymorphous perversity came from a variety of traditions. See, for instance:

Baldwin, James. (1998). "Freaks and the American Ideal of Manhood", in Toni Morrison (ed.) *James Baldwin: Collected Essays*. New York: Library of America, pp. 814–829.

Firestone, Shulamith. (1970). *The Dialectic of Sex: The Case for Feminist Revolution*. New York: William Morrow.

Mieli, Mario. (2018). *Towards a Gay Communism: Elements of a Homosexual Critique*, David Fernbach and Evan Calder Williams (trans.). London: Pluto Press.

Science fiction is a great source for thinking about conceptual gaps, gender, and the potential for misunderstanding (and diplomatic issues!) that can come from the interaction of societies with radically different understandings of gender. Perhaps the best example of this is Ursula K. Le Guin's masterpiece, *The Left Hand of Darkness.*

Le Guin, Ursula K. (2000). *The Left Hand of Darkness*. New York: Ace Books.

7

THE TRANS THEORY TRADITION

After what we're looked at so far in this book, you might be wondering about the history of this field. Did trans philosophy just pop into existence in recent years? Clearly not. But where did it come from? To answer this question, we're going to have to do some history of philosophy! So where does contemporary trans philosophy come from? Well, there's perhaps as many sources for contemporary trans philosophy as there are trans philosophers! However, there are a couple of scholarly traditions that have had an outsize influence on trans philosophy and have shaped the field as we know it today: *feminist philosophy* and *trans theory*.

Feminist philosophy is an incredibly rich tradition in its own right, and we won't examine it in detail here, because it would be worth a whole book on its own! But it's worth noting that many, if not most, contemporary academic trans philosophers were supervised by feminist philosophers, feminist philosophers have contributed greatly to trans philosophy itself, and it is in feminist journals like *Hypatia* and *Feminist Philosophy Quarterly* that much transgender philosophy is published. As such, many of the political and methodological concerns of feminist philosophers have been inherited by transgender philosophers. We saw some of that influence in our discussion of the metaphysics of gender in Chapter 1.

DOI: 10.4324/9781003502944-8

The other key ancestor of most contemporary trans philosophy, and the one we'll spend the rest of this chapter looking at, is a tradition known as 'trans theory'. This name might sound a bit confusing: isn't 'theory' a synonym for 'philosophy', or at least isn't theory something very much like philosophy? If so, what distinguishes trans theory from trans philosophy? The answer is, to my mind at least, *not much*. I would happily characterise everything we'll go on to discuss in this chapter as philosophy! However, the label 'trans theory' tends to be applied to the particular historical tradition in trans thought that we'll discuss in this chapter, so it's a useful label for us to use here. Part of the reason for this naming convention is that what people call 'trans theory' was rarely, if ever, done in philosophy departments. If discussed in universities at all, trans thought of this kind was largely undertaken in North American literature, language, and communications departments. In such departments, more philosophical work tends to be called 'literary theory', 'high theory', or simply just 'theory'. Given that professional philosophers were late to the party in discussing this tradition, the name 'trans theory' has stuck.

Whatever we call it, it's clear that contemporary trans philosophy owes a great deal to the work done in this tradition. The ways of thinking about trans issues developed in trans theory have gone on to shape the work done in contemporary trans philosophy in important ways – the thinkers here often serve as direct interlocutors to be responded to or as implicit figures who have framed the debates at the heart of trans philosophy. Contemporary trans philosophers aren't just responding to Simone de Beauvoir, David Hume, and Sally Haslanger. They're also in dialogue with Susan Stryker, Judith Butler, and Sandy Stone: figures in the trans theory tradition that we'll explore in this chapter.

One final note before we begin: whilst in this chapter we'll only look at trans theory up until the turn of the millennium, you shouldn't read that as suggesting that trans theory no longer exists or has been supplanted by trans philosophy! More recent trans theory has gone in a variety of different directions, often with a greater emphasis on how being trans interacts with issues of race, disability, and sexuality – and you can find some of these works in the recommended further readings section.

THE TRANSSEXUAL EMPIRE

Some of the first forays into the field that will become known as 'trans theory' come from trans thinkers' responses to exclusionary feminist theory in the 1980s. Perhaps the most famous exchange here is that between Janice Raymond and Sandy Stone. Raymond's book, *The Transsexual Empire: The Making of the She-Male*, expresses a forthright cultural feminist position on trans people, focusing on trans women.[1] Cultural feminism is one branch of radical feminism, which is distinguished from other types of radical feminism by its claim that, "the enemy of women is not merely a social system or economic institution or set of backward beliefs but masculinity itself and in some cases male biology".[2] This tends to result in a position whereby maleness and femaleness are essentially different – not something that can be bridged or transitioned between.

Raymond argues that trans women are either the dupes, or willing agents of, patriarchy and male supremacy. For Raymond, those men (to her mind) who pretend to be women via crossdressing and medical intervention are deeply offensive on several levels. At a base level, trans women fetishise and reinforce stereotypes of femininity, mocking 'real' women as a cruel parody. More pressingly, according to Raymond, such pretenders also seek to infiltrate the feminist movement, undermining it from the inside. Infamously, Raymond's most extreme claim is that trans women rape women's bodies in transitioning.[3]

The trans-exclusionary nature of feminist movements in the 1970s and 1980s is often overstated. As Emily Cousens has recently demonstrated, trans people, especially trans women, were central to the development of many parts of radical feminism, and many radical feminists of the period were supportive of trans people.[4] Raymond certainly was expressing a view that was shared (at least in broad outlines) by many cultural and radical feminists from this time, but there were plenty of radical feminist communities that saw trans women as women. One such community was Olivia Records – a lesbian feminist record label where the trans woman Sandy Stone worked as a sound engineer.

Stone gives us a direct response to Raymond in her famous essay "The Empire Strikes Back: A Posttranssexual Manifesto".[5] Stone had been singled out by Raymond in *The Transsexual Empire,* with Raymond accusing Stone of undermining Olivia Records with her "masculine behavior" and "male energy".[6] The acrimonious dispute over Stone's role at Olivia Records culminated in Stone leaving Olivia Records, despite the support of its collective, following the extensive harassment of Stone and death threats from a lesbian separatist organisation known as the Gorgons.[7] In "The Empire Strikes Back", Stone emphasises the plurality of transness. There is no single mode of life that all trans people, even all trans women, all share. Sure, there are trans women who see themselves as embodying a stereotypical femininity, passing as cisgender, largely in response to a medical establishment that demands such femininity if they are to access medical care. However, there are modes of trans life that reject attempts to 'fit in', and which push back against any demand from wider society that one passes. Raymond, argues Stone, assumes that all trans women are of the former camp.

One thing we might think about Stone's argument is that it concedes too much to Raymond. It seems to accept that many trans women are particularly responsible for reinforcing stereotypes of femininity and that they hence are in some sense problematic. Stone's essay concludes, for instance, with the claim that the radical trans community attempts to recruit those trans people who are interested in passing, into a project of undoing gender entirely. You might think that there are better ways to respond to Raymond – some of which we discussed in Chapter 4. Stone also thinks that passing trans people fail to take responsibility for "*all* of their history", denying their differences from cisgender people.[8] This is troublesome, suggests Stone, as it impedes a project of a radical transformation of society away from an oppressive binary gender system. Against all this, I can't help but wonder whether there are possibilities for a radical transgender politics that begin from a demand to be seen as a woman or a man. Must all trans people have a gender along the lines of Dembroff's critical gender kinds or else count as reinforcing stereotypes and a binary gender system? You might think there's a space for a form of trans politics that doesn't answer this question with a 'yes', especially if one thinks that feminism isn't also undermined by feminists who think of themselves as women.

STRYKER'S MONSTER

Stone was not the only influential theorist working at this time. Another key figure from this moment is Susan Stryker, whose performance piece "My Words to Victor Frankenstein Above the Village of Chamounix" has become a foundational text in trans studies. Stryker conceives of the position of trans people in cis society as being akin to that of Frankenstein's monster in Mary Shelley's novel. Stigmatised, marginalised, and excluded from mainstream social life, trans people are often treated as monstrous. Sometimes this treatment is implicit, expressed through phenomena like shunning, but as Stryker documents, there are plenty of examples of cisgender people literally calling trans people monsters. For instance, Stryker quotes one letter written to the editor of a San Francisco gay/lesbian periodical, where the author attacks a trans lesbian that had recently given a public talk:

> When an estrogenated man with breasts loves a woman, that is not lesbianism, that is mutilated perversion. [This individual] is not a threat to the lesbian community, he is an outrage to us. He is not a lesbian, he is a mutant man, a self-made freak, a deformity, an insult. He deserves a slap in the face.[9]

Of course, treating trans people as monsters often has terrible effects. But Stryker wants to suggest that trans people could *reclaim* the image of the monster.

What is it to 'reclaim' something in this context? Well, the classic example here is the reclamation of slurs. Take, for instance, the N-word. The N-word has, for centuries, been used as a slur against Black people, demeaning them and treating them as less than human. However, especially in the latter half of the 20th century, African-American people began to reframe the N-word, using it in artistic performance and community building. By using the word positively and on their own terms, Black people are able to take a degree of control over the slur. Whilst hardly an uncontroversial practice, similar reclamation projects have been undertaken by a variety of oppressed groups. Feminists, for instance, have often been keen to positively identify with 'witch' and 'bitch', whilst gay men have in some contexts reclaimed 'fag' and 'fairy'. Of course, such slurs are still horribly offensive when used *about* members of such groups by outsiders. However, when used in self-description, these words can be powerful symbols of shared identity and pride.

Stryker offers us a similar idea, but about the derogatory social category or image of *the monster*. They write, "I want to lay claim to the dark power of my monstrous identity without using it as a weapon against others or being wounded by it myself".[10] What is this 'dark power'? Well, one might think that there are a few different 'powers' that the image of the monster offers to trans people. On the one hand, you might think that it offers a way for trans people to think of themselves as powerful, so powerful, in fact, that society is terrified of them! This might offer trans people confidence and pride in the face of an oppressive society. On the other, Stryker sees identifying with the image of the monster as a way of legitimating and seeing as acceptable the anger that a trans person might feel towards an exclusionary cisgender society, in what they call 'transgender rage'. Perhaps most interestingly, however, is a further power that the figure of the monster offers: for Stryker, to be a transgender monster is to be a herald of change, a figure who arrives to tell the world that a great upheaval is on the way:

> "Monster" is derived from the Latin noun monstrum, "divine portent", itself formed on the root of the verb monere, "to warn". It came to refer to living things of anomalous shape or structure, or to fabulous creatures like the sphinx who were composed of strikingly incongruous parts, because the ancients considered the appearance of such beings to be a sign of some impending supernatural event. Monsters, like angels, functioned as messengers and heralds of the extraordinary. They served to announce impending revelation, saying, in effect, "Pay attention; something of profound importance is happening".[11]

Whilst the monster in general might herald all sorts of things, Stryker suggests that (at least at the time that they were writing in the 1990s) the transgender monster heralds a particular kind of revolution. This great change, according to Stryker, is a profound change in how society understands sex, gender, and the body. Rather than thinking of ourselves as natural, a revolution in our thinking will occur, such that everyone begins to think of themselves as constructed in some important sense:

> Hearken unto me, fellow creatures. I who have dwelt in a form unmatched with my desire, I whose flesh has become an assemblage of incongruous anatomical parts, I who achieve the similitude of a natural body only through an unnatural process, I offer you this warning: the Nature you bedevil me with is a lie. Do not trust it to protect you from what I represent, for it is a fabrication that cloaks the groundlessness of the privilege you seek to maintain for yourself at my expense. You are as constructed as me; the same anarchic Womb has birthed us both. I call upon you to investigate your nature as I have been compelled to confront mine. I challenge you to risk abjection and flourish as well as have I. Heed my words, and you may well discover the seams and sutures in yourself.[12]

How is this revolution supposed to occur? Well, Styker begins from trans people who undertake medical interventions to shape their bodies. Their bodies have, according to Stryker, been quite literally constructed by biomedical science, just like Frankenstein's monster! However, once we see this, we quickly come to realise that this construction doesn't just happen in the gender clinic: virtually everyone's body will be changed at some point or other through medical science, whether via a knee replacement, a tablet to suppress an immune response, or a procedure to remove a tooth. Moreover, why should we just consider *medical* construction? Stryker thinks that we will soon realise that our bodies are profoundly shaped and made by our culture at large. We'll think about this claim in a little more detail in the next section in discussing the work of Judith Butler.

Is Stryker right that "To encounter the transsexual body, to apprehend a transgendered consciousness articulating itself, is to risk a revelation of the constructedness of the natural order"?[13] That is, are they right that trans people are heralds of a revolution in the way we think about gender, sex and the body? One might be sceptical. Even if Stryker is correct that trans people demonstrate that gender and the body aren't natural, and that this *should* mean that cisgender people begin to think of themselves as non-natural too, you might think that cisgender people might just refuse to accept this. That is, one cognitive defence mechanism against this troubling challenge to an ingrained set of beliefs is to simply deny that it also applies to cisgender people. Trans people, in this way of thinking, are monsters. The defensive cisgender person might simply think or assume that 'trans people, as monsters, are fundamentally *different from us* and hence, even if they are constructed by culture or biomedical science, that tells us nothing about us normal cisgender people'.

However, perhaps we shouldn't be so pessimistic about Stryker's predictions, given that there have been large changes in how so many people think about gender in the past 30 or so years. Sure, there are plenty of defensive cisgender people, but nevertheless, the increased cultural prominence of transgender people has heralded big changes in the social landscape and how gender is treated. Things haven't changed in exactly the way Stryker thought they would, but they definitely have shifted! For instance, during my own youth, I was educated under so-called 'Section 28', which prohibited teaching that queer relationships were acceptable in British schools. Now, LGBTQ+ school clubs are commonplace in the UK, and the cultural acceptance of queer people has been fundamentally reshaped for the better – though not, of course, without backlash from reactionary groups.

BUTLER, QUEER THEORY, NAMASTE, PROSSER

Many of the themes in Stryker's work are shared with perhaps the most famous work in philosophy from this period: Judith Butler's *Gender Trouble*.[14] Butler was not out as nonbinary at the time, but their book was to become foundational for much trans and queer activism in the 1990s, in addition to revolutionising feminist philosophy and helping to found the field known as 'queer theory'. A proper summation of this book and its inheritors would go well beyond the scope of this present volume![15] However, it's worth saying a few things about the sort of metaphysical and political positions that emerged in the wake of its publication.

Butler argues that gender is 'performative'. That is, gender is constituted through repeated stylised performances that reference earlier performances and norms of behaviour. So, when a woman wears a wedding dress to get married, she is engaging in a practice of stylised behaviour and gets counted as a woman (in part) because other women have also worn that type of dress before when getting married. Her performance cites all of those previous performances, solidifying her own status as a woman, and in turn she helps to solidify the particular sorts of roles that women 'should' take in society via the example she sets. Of course, actually performing womanhood requires more than just this one aspect of one (admittedly very important) day's dress. Crucial to Butler's position is that maintaining one's gender involves repeated and consistent activity, creating the (false) impression that one is *really* or *essentially* a woman, underneath these varied performances.

One of Butler's more radical claims is that *sex* is socially constructed, in addition to gender. That might sound surprising: normally people say that gender is a social construct, but not sex! After all, aren't things like penises, chromosomes, and hormones biological, not social? Butler's strategy is to argue that gender is prior to sex, and that therefore society's insistence on a binary sex system is an effect of society's insistence on a binary gender system. So, in being an effect of the gender social structure, sex as a binary must also be social, even if bodies themselves are biological.

How is this argument supposed to work? Well, we have a society that insists on a rigid and patriarchal gender binary, with different roles, aesthetics, and hierarchical positions for men and women. This set of social constructs that we call 'gender' infects all aspects of our lives, and requires justification against those who would critique it. After all, a woman stuck in such a society might demand to know why she has to do housework but not her brother. A sex binary is therefore used in such a society to justify the gender binary: you have to do the housework because you're naturally different to your brother, and this is women's natural position in society. So: the gender binary produces the sex binary in order to defend and justify itself. Sometimes this even extends to the literal construction of new genitals: in many jurisdictions intersex children with ambiguous genitalia are operated on in order to give them unambiguously male or female genitalia.

So: according to Butler, society features gender and sex binaries that are tightly connected. To be a man in such a society is to have a particular set of genitalia that one has had since birth and to fulfil male gender roles. Now, this potentially leaves room for political action to undermine such a patriarchal society. If one can find a way to undermine the supposedly tight connection between sex and gender, one might think that we could undermine the patriarchy. As such, queer political philosophers and activists that drew on Butler's work tended to think of trans people as potentially radical political actors. After all, who better to demonstrate that sex does not naturally determine one's gender or place in society than a trans person who has rejected the sex that they were assigned at birth?

Thus, the queer theory and activism that developed out of this tradition were centred around projects of gendered play, parody, and drag, trying to disrupt the supposedly neat binaries of wider society. Here, trans people are inherently politically radical, destabilising patriarchy, undermining rigid roles. Trans people, in this account, demonstrate that gender is ultimately a fiction, with some thinkers like Jack Halberstam going so far as to argue that gender being a fiction implies that being a trans man or trans woman doesn't actually make sense:

> the referent becomes less and less clear (and more and more queer). We are all cross-dressers, but where are we crossing from or to what? There is no 'other' side, no 'opposite' sex, no natural divide to be spanned by surgery, by disguise, by passing. We all pass or we don't. . . . There are no transsexuals.[16]

This, you might think, is an odd position to end up in! Queer theorists, beginning from a purportedly radical and trans-inclusive perspective, seem to have reached the conclusion that gender is a fiction and that trans people don't really exist. You might think that this is hardly much better than the cultural feminists like Raymond who accused trans women of being men.

Two trans theorists who made this sort of argument against queer theory were Jay Prosser and Viviane Namaste. Whilst they wrote separately, I have argued that they are worth considering together, given that their critiques are remarkably aligned, and that they were writing at around the same time.[17] Prosser and Namaste each argued that the queer theorist fails to do justice to trans people *as actual people*. Central to this line of argument is queer theory abstracts away from the realities of trans people and our lives, focusing instead on the transgender *figure*. This transgender figure is not a real person, or even a generalisation about trans people, but is rather the *idea* of a person who transitions genders, given a particular theoretical model of society. Prosser and Namaste instead urge us to refocus on trans people themselves and the lives that they live.[18]

Remember that the queer theorist that Prosser and Namaste objects to has a model of society whereby mainstream gendered social life is justified by a supposed connection to a 'natural' sex. That you supposedly have to become a wife, settle down, and have two kids is justified in mainstream society by the claim that this is what is natural for women as a sex to do. Trans people, according to the queer theorist, are inherently radical: they demonstrate that the connection between sex and the gendered way one lives is not a necessary one. One could have been born with a penis and yet still live one's life as a woman and do womanly things. For this sort of queer theorist, the transgender figure undermines the foundations of a society that is organised around a supposedly natural sex and its connection to gender, demonstrating that it was all a fiction.

However, this just doesn't seem to capture how many trans people themselves relate to sex and society. For many, if not most, trans people, their sex isn't a justification that they want to reveal to be fictitious: sex is all too real. The experience of dysphoria is, for many trans people, the experience of a sexed body as wrong, distressing, or otherwise unpleasant. *If only* it could just be demonstrated to be a fiction and imagined away! No, instead, many trans people undertake hormonal and surgical interventions in order to change their sexed features. Moreover, this process most often is not just about destroying undesirable aspects of the old body: it's about building a new one. Sex here is literally constructed, but it's not fictitious or unreal – it's a vital way of overcoming dysphoria and building a new identity in transition.

The complex reality of trans life, and how trans people engage with their sexed bodies, has, argue Prosser and Namaste, been idealised away in the queer theory tradition. Instead, of being treated as real people, trans people are treated as radical ideal figures who have the power to undermine an oppressive society: "transsexual and transgendered people are reduced to the merely figural: rhetorical tropes and discursive levers".[19] Prosser and Namaste instead push us to return to actual trans people.

PRECIADO AGAINST BEING BORING

One not particularly charitable reading of Namaste and Prosser is that in their view, trans people are pretty darn *boring*. We're just ordinary people, struggling to get by in a world that seems to be offended by our very existence. There seemed to be good reason for Namaste and Prosser to insist on our ordinariness: queer theorists had used a 'figure of transgender' to insist that trans people were radical political actors in ways that seemed quite alien to actual transgender people. Moreover, you might think that insisting that we're *just ordinary people* is itself a useful political tactic. If it were possible to persuade wider society that we're just like them, you might think this would go some way towards reducing violence and discrimination against trans people.

However, there are a couple of reasons to resist the idea that we should think of trans people as just boring normal people. One is that, in an important sense, when a trans person transitions, they are doing something that challenges the dominant gender ideology that we saw Dembroff discuss in Chapter 1. Transgender people who transition act in ways that disrupt our ordinary ways of organising and thinking about gender. Someone who does this can hardly be described as boring and normal – at least in our current society!

Another reason to challenge 'trans normalcy' is that you might think that it is an unwise political strategy. If our attempt to end discrimination and violence against trans people is based on the idea that we can persuade cisgender people that we are just like them, and that we can fit into polite society with them, then you might find it a very difficult task. Moreover, even if we do manage to persuade cisgender society that transgender people are 'normal', you might worry that there will still be plenty of people who society still regards as abnormal and hence permissible to discriminate against – some of whom will be trans. Even if polite society is happy to accept most trans people as 'normal', you might worry that without a more radical change to society, discrimination against sex workers, Black people, disabled people, and so on will still exist – and of course many of these people will also be transgender. What's worse, if some transgender people have been fully assimilated into the mainstream, you might think that such discrimination is in some way tacitly endorsed by the 'normal' trans people.

Finally, is normalcy desirable? For many trans people, transitioning and 'fitting in' with cisgender society is a goal. However, for many others, transitioning was never about fitting in. Instead, it is about finding new ways of living gender beyond the narrow model given by dominant gender ideology. And, as we'll see in the next chapter, *lots* of trans people want to radically reshape society. So, even if we think that Namaste and Prosser were right in their criticisms of queer theory, is there a way of reclaiming the idea that trans people *can* be radical political actors against normalcy?

Paul Preciado offers us one vision of how this might be achieved. Preciado utterly rejects any call for trans liberation through assimilation to the normal, writing that we should instead embrace 'countersexuality':

> Against the reformist and integrationist legal agenda of lesbian, gay, bisexual, trans (LGBT) identity movements, countersexuality proposes a new configuration of the relationship between desire and body, between technology and consciousness. Against a fight for recognition and representation of identities according to traditional democratic means (voting, changing the law, etc.), I suggest radically experimenting with new practices of collective sexual emancipation and sexual self-government.[20]

For Preciado, most sexuality in contemporary cisgender society merely repeats a narrow script of male-female desire, according to which certain bodies are defined as having certain functions that must be followed: the male body must have a penis which must become erect at the appropriate time, must ejaculate in the female body and so on.[21] The countersexual, by contrast, seeks to experiment with bodies and technologies so as to undermine these scripts.

What do these experiments look like? Well, they can involve reworking sexual practices in ways that undermine traditional scripts, not least in BDSM, anal play, and the use of dildos.[22] For Preciado, pegging your boyfriend is a radical political act! However, Preciado also thinks that bodily transformations of the sort undertaken by trans people can also undermine traditional scripts of sexuality, subverting traditional narratives of what it is to be a man, for instance. In so doing, Preciado thinks we can undermine the idea that there is a natural gender binary and heterosexual sexuality, demonstrating quite literally how gender and sexuality can be constructed. This set of practices is something that Preciado follows through on himself. In his *Testo Junkie*, he recounts his various sexual and gender practices through which he attempts to rewrite dominant ideas about sexuality and gender. Most strikingly, he describes his experiments with taking testosterone he has sourced from a "gender hacker" friend (rather than going through a doctor-approved medical transition).[23]

Wait a minute – how is this any different from queer theory's treatment of trans people as radical political actors? Preciado thinks that seemingly any trans person is going to be inherently radical, undermining traditional sexual and gender scripts. So, potentially Preciado's position is just as vulnerable to Prosser and Namaste's arguments as the queer theorist's position! However, note that Preciado is doing something slightly different than the queer theorist. Where the queer theorist relied on an ideal figure of transgender, abstracted away from actual trans people, Preciado is instead suggesting a set of practices that can be done by actual trans people (and indeed anyone interested in challenging gender normalcy).

In queer theory, trans people tended to be treated as radical figures because they supposedly demonstrated the fictitious nature of sex, when so many trans people in fact dealt with the material reality of sex on an everyday basis. Meanwhile, for Preciado, sex is something that is very real but also very malleable. We can act upon our bodies to change them, making something new that radically challenges the idea that sex, sexuality, and gender are binary and fixed. In so doing, Preciado hopes we can open up new ways of living. Instead of assimilating into normal society, we have the opportunity to challenge it through remaking our bodies and rethinking how we relate to one another.

With this said, you might still be sceptical. Will these sorts of interventions on our bodies and sexual practices really be enough to overthrow existing cisgender society and bring about a new world? You might worry that society will simply act to treat it as an acceptable exception, regarding radicals like Preciado as simply weird and with no implications for how the cisgender majority of people should start living their lives. Or worse, cisgender society might act to stamp out this challenge, restricting access to hormones, passing laws against crossdressing, and otherwise criminalising these radical individuals. You might think that instead of these acts of resistance against cisgender society that take place at the individual and interpersonal level, we instead need a broader movement that can truly challenge cisgender society and its dominant gender ideology. In the next chapter, we'll see how some transgender philosophers have thought about this political challenge.

NOTES

1 Raymond, Janice. (1994). *The Transsexual Empire: The Making of the She-Male*. New York and London: Teachers Press.

2 Alcoff, Linda Martin. (1988). "Cultural Feminism versus Post-Structuralism: The Identity Crisis in Feminist Theory". *Signs* 13(3): 408.

3 Raymond, *The Transsexual Empire*, 104.

4 Cousens, Emily. (2023). *Trans Feminist Epistemologies in the US Second Wave*. New York and London: Palgrave Macmillan.

5 Stone, Sandy. (1993). "The Empire Strikes Back: A Posttranssexual Manifesto". *sandystone.com*. https://sandystone.com/empire-strikes-back.pdf

6 Raymond, *Transsexual Empire*, 101–102.

7 See Male, Andrew. (2020). "'Our Sound Engineer got a Death Threat': How Lesbian Label Olivia Shook up Music". *The Guardian*. https://www.theguardian.com/music/2020/jul/19/lesbian-record-label-olivia-linda-tillery-californian-feminists-death-threat-music. For more on Olivia, see Berson, Ginny. (2020). *Olivia on the Record: A Radical Experiment in Women's Music*. California: Aunt Lute Books.

8 Stone, "Empire Strikes Back", 16.
9 Mikuteit, Debbie, quoted in Stryker, Susan. (1994). "My Words to Victor Frankenstein Above the Village of Chamounix: Performing Transgender Rage". *GLQ* 1(3): 239.
10 Stryker, "My Words to Victor Frankenstein", 240.
11 Stryker, "My Words to Victor Frankenstein".
12 Stryker, "My Words to Victor Frankenstein", 240–241.
13 Stryker, "My Words to Victor Frankenstein", 250.
14 Butler, Judith. (1999). *Gender Trouble: Tenth Anniversary Edition*. Routledge.
15 Butler's work has been especially influential in the fields of performance studies and science and technology studies.
16 Halberstam, Jack. (1994). "F2M: The Making of Female Masculinity", in L. Doan (ed.) *The Lesbian Postmodern*. New York: Columbia University Press, pp. 210–228.
17 I explore Namaste and Prosser's work at greater length and further argue that they should be seen as working in the tradition of nonideal theory in Cull, Matthew J. (2025). "Ideal Theory, Literary Theory, Whither Transfeminism?", in Hilkje Charlotte Hänel and Johanna M. Müller (eds.) *The Routledge Handbook of Non-Ideal Theory*. New York: Routledge, pp. 246–258.
18 See Namaste, Viviane. (2000). *Invisible Lives: The Erasure of Transsexual and Transgendered People*. Chicago and London: University of Chicago Press and Prosser, Jay. (1998). *Second Skins: The Body Narratives of Transsexuality*. New York: Columbia University Press.
19 Namaste, *Invisible Lives*, 51–52.
20 Preciado, Paul. (2000/2018). *Countersexual Manifesto*, Kevin Gerry Dunn (trans.). New York: Columbia University Press, p. 14.
21 Preciado, *Countersexual Manifesto*, 10.
22 Preciado, *Countersexual Manifesto*, 29.
23 Preciado, Paul B. (2013). *Testo Junkie: Sex, Drugs, and Biopolitics in the Pharmacopornographic Era*. New York: Feminist Press, p. 55.

RECOMMENDATIONS FOR FURTHER READING

In addition to the works already cited in this chapter, those wanting to think more about the topics raised here might like to take a look at the following:

Feminist philosophy and trans theory are hardly the only major influences on contemporary trans philosophy. In the next chapter we'll look at the influence of Marxist and anarchist thought on trans philosophy, but some other key influences include the Black radical tradition and psychoanalysis. The discussion of these in the *Transgender Studies Quarterly* issue on 'The Issue of

Blackness', along with some of the works of Paul Preciado and Trish Salah, are good places to start on each of these, respectively:

Ellison, Treva, Green, Kai M., Richardson, Matt and Snorton, C. Riley (eds.). (2017). "The Issue of Blackness". *Transgender Studies Quarterly* 4(2).

Preciado, Paul B. (2021). *Can the Monster Speak?*, Frank Wynne (trans.). London: Fitzcarraldo.

Salah, Trish. (2017). "What Does Tiresias Want?". *Transgender Studies Quarterly* 4(3–4): 632–638.

One very exciting and radical figure in the trans theory tradition is Riki Wilchins, whose oppositional approach to gender remains incredibly influential today:

Wilchins, Riki. (1997). *Read My Lips: Sexual Subversion and the End of Gender.* New York: Magnus Books.

Butler's later work has developed in ways that are less vulnerable to the sorts of criticism developed by Prosser and Namaste, developing a version of queer theory that takes the body seriously rather than treating it as a mere figure:

Butler, Judith. (2004). *Undoing Gender.* Abingdon: Routledge.

Transgender Studies Quarterly has also seen some interesting discussion of trans theory as an enterprise. Writing there, Andrea Long and has sounded a sceptical note about whether trans theory is a successful research program that has been able to break from queer theory:

Chu, Andrea Long and Harsin Drager, Emmett. (2019). "After Trans Studies". *TSQ* 6(1): 103–116.

Early trans theory didn't *only* happen in North America. Prosser, for instance, was working in the UK when *Second Skins* was published, whilst Preciado has worked in France and Spain for some time. Other sources of British trans theory include Kate More and Stephen Whittle, who collaborated on a collected volume together:

More, Kate and Whittle, Stephen (eds.). (1999). *Reclaiming Genders: Transsexual Grammars at the Fin de Siècle.* London and New York: Cassell.

More recent trans theory has gone in a variety of different and exciting directions. A couple of figures that readers might enjoy engaging with include micha cárdenas and Cameron Awkward-Rich:

Awkward-Rich, Cameron. (2022). *The Terrible We: Thinking with Trans Maladjustment.* Durham: Duke University Press.

cárdenas, micha. (2016). "Pregnancy: Reproductive Futures in Trans of Color Feminism". *TSQ* 3(1–2): 48–57.

8

POLITICAL PHILOSOPHY

Politics has, of course, been central to many of the topics in this book. Political concerns have shaped how trans philosophers have explored issues in metaphysics, epistemology, and beyond. The trans theory tradition was especially attuned to political issues, deeply concerned with the place of trans people in society. However, what have transgender philosophers had to say about *political philosophy*? That is, what have transgender philosophers had to say about traditional questions such as those regarding the distribution of rights and goods in society, the authority and nature of the state, and the ways that our collective lives ought to be lived?

One curious feature of trans political philosophy is the relative absence of thinkers who might be characterised as liberal, conservative, or otherwise 'centrist'. In mainstream political philosophy, debates have largely been dominated by debates between different parts of the political centre ground. Meanwhile transgender political thought has largely involved debates among various left-wing positions. In this chapter we'll investigate how and why trans political philosophy has departed from mainstream political philosophy. We'll also explore where and why trans political philosophers differ from one another.

DOI: 10.4324/9781003502944-9

MAINSTREAM POLITICAL PHILOSOPHY

If you've ever studied political philosophy before, you'll have come across some 20th-century figures like John Rawls and Robert Nozick, or perhaps some earlier figures like John Locke and Immanuel Kant. Such figures have dominated debates in political philosophy from their own time to the present. Whilst these figures have important differences between them, the mainstream tradition that they have inspired features a number of assumptions which all sides in the debate tend to agree on:

- Our philosophical analyses should begin from the assumption that there are individuals who are bearers of rights.
- That there ought to be states and that states along with individuals must be at the centre of our analyses.
- A, or perhaps even *the*, central question of political philosophy is justifying the state's authority and laws.
- Capitalism is the best way to organise the production and distribution of goods.
- Injustices like racism and sexism are to be explained in terms of individual biases and prejudices, not in terms of social structures.
- Historical injustices like colonialism may be unfortunate, but they do not factor into how society should be organised *today*.

People in the mainstream debate might disagree on exactly what rights individuals have and how competing demands between individuals are to be balanced. However, they generally accept that individuals with rights are to be at the heart of our investigation, along with how these individuals relate to states. Similarly, whilst such liberals and conservatives might disagree on how much redistribution is justified, they all nevertheless agree that capitalism is the background condition against which that redistribution takes place. Rawls and Nozick might disagree on how much power the state is supposed to have, but they both agree that there should at least be something we call a state.

This consensus in American and European political philosophy matches a consensus in the politics of most of Europe, Canada, and the United States. Take the example of the United Kingdom, where (as elsewhere in the world) the various mainstream political parties share a political centre ground. The British Labour and Conservative parties might disagree on how big the welfare state is or what sorts of restrictions the state should put on individual enterprise, but they both agree that capitalism is the best way to organise the economy and that the state must have the power to intervene on individual action in at least some circumstances.

It's not obvious which way causation runs here. Does political philosophy determine what politics looks like? Well, if you listen to certain politicians, you might think so. Former British Prime Minister Tony Blair claimed that he was influenced by John Rawls, and politicians from many parties cite classic liberal philosophers such as John Locke as key figures in shaping their politics. But you might also think that causation runs in the opposite direction: political philosophers are surely influenced by their political contexts when developing their ideas. We might also think that which ideas get published and come to gain influence might also be determined by the politics of the day. In some cases, we even see direct interventions into philosophy by politicians, as in McCarthy's purges of left-wing thinkers from US academia.[1] But perhaps we don't have to come down on one side or the other here: plausibly, political philosophy and politics itself shape one another. We'll return to the significance of this connection in the next section.

WHY RADICAL POLITICS?

Transgender philosophers have overwhelmingly departed from this centre ground. In one way or another, they have rejected assumptions of the mainstream debate. Instead, they have adopted political positions derived from a number of alternative sources, including Marxism, anarchism, the Black radical tradition, and accelerationism. Before we look in any more detail at these positions, however, we should first ask: Why have transgender political philosophers almost universally rejected mainstream centrist political philosophy?

Now, there are probably as many reasons for trans philosophers adopting radical political views as there are trans philosophers.

However, there are a couple of sociological factors which are worth noting. The first is that trans people, and by extension trans philosophers, tend to be marginalised by mainstream society. The second is that trans people have found alternative spaces for philosophical discussion in community and online spaces. Let's think about why each factor might predispose trans philosophers away from liberal political philosophy in turn.

First, the marginalisation faced by trans people. This marginalisation is both social and economic. Trans people often face ostracisation from important social institutions such as the family, transphobic bullying, and even violence. Meanwhile, trans people are more likely to be precariously employed or unemployed than their cis counterparts. Now, whatever one thinks of the way we currently organise our societies and our economies, it's pretty clear that trans people aren't being treated particularly well. As such, any set of philosophical positions that (broadly speaking) suggests that society is working in a (more or less) good way as things stand is likely going to be unattractive to trans philosophers. After all, such a set of philosophical positions would run contrary to their own experience or discount it as not mattering when it comes to judging what counts as a good society.

Liberal and conservative positions are, as we noted previously, something like the philosophy of the status quo. Whilst they might have minor quibbles over the details of how exactly society should be run, mainstream political philosophers broadly take it that the liberal capitalist state *is more or less how things should be*. It is no wonder then, that trans people, whose existence on the margins of that society is so fraught with violence and poverty, would think that a different way of philosophising about society is needed.

Second, let's think about the philosophical communities that trans people have developed. Trans people in philosophy departments have, until very recently, been extremely rare creatures (they are still rare, mind!). As such, when trans people wanted to discuss politics and philosophy, they rarely had access to the resources and debates that were happening inside the academy. Instead, trans people turned to their own local groups, specialist periodicals, zines, and online spaces.[2] In these alternative spaces for discussion, trans people have been able to develop philosophical views that diverge from the mainstream. Whilst they lacked the resources of the academy, such spaces were not hemmed in by the hegemony of liberal political philosophy, where anything not citing Rawls would be laughed out of the room.

None of this suggests that trans people always and uniformly go for more radical political views (and indeed in the further readings, I point to some of the few liberal trans political philosophers), but it does help us to explain why trans people are more likely to be on the far left (or occasionally far right) than their cis counterparts.

TRANSGENDER ANARCHISM

Of course, as noted earlier in this chapter, trans political philosophy tends to come from positions of marginalisation, exclusion, and dispossession at the hands of wider society. Under such circumstances, the idea that we should *tear it all down* looks like it might have some appeal. Hence, there has been much exploration of the notion of *abolition*, especially amongst trans philosophers influenced by anarchism and the Black radical tradition. In the last chapter we explored *gender* abolitionist positions, but here we'll focus on work that employs a broader notion of abolition. This broader notion of abolition suggests that it is not just gender that should be abolished: rather, most of how we currently organise society should be abolished, including prisons, states, and capitalism. Nat Raha and Mijke Van Der Drift, in their *Trans Femme Futures*, give us an excellent example of this kind of work.[3] Raha and Van Der Drift argue that trans liberation cannot occur via institutions. Instead, we ought to seek liberation by abolishing institutions and forming alternative modes of social organisation.

For Raha and Van Der Drift, institutions are things like states, universities, corporations, legal systems, and so on. Institutions are instruments of control, and they usually operate through violence: locking people out, locking people up, and threatening to dispossess people of their assets. Such forms of social organisation, they argue, cannot be salvaged. Many NGOs that purport to advocate for trans people call for inclusion within mainstream institutions or call for trans rights, which might entitle trans people to improved treatment by such institutions. However, Raha and Van Der Drift agitate against any political strategy aimed at inclusion of this sort.

It might seem surprising that some trans philosophers would argue against fighting for trans rights. After all, one might think, what's wrong with more rights? Sure, many institutions traditionally only gave rights to straight White men and excluded women, people of colour, and gay people from having rights, and that was morally wrong. However (for the most part), such institutions have now extended rights to these groups. One might therefore think that whilst it's a shame that many such institutions haven't yet extended the same rights to trans people, surely the inclusion of trans people would be the next step in rectifying injustice against those excluded from traditional rights frameworks.

Raha and Van Der Drift disagree, as they see rights as a form of control:

> We are hesitant to rely on institutional and legal reforms for social change. Institutions curb our movements. Institutions function to stabilise the world, erecting fences to enable the control of an environment by management. Liberal institutions emerge from European Enlightenment philosophies [sic] ideas of knowledge and individual agency. In these theories, the boundaries of knowledge contain what can be controlled, while everything else is excluded as 'chaos'. To be unknown is to have no place in the structure, which entails not having access to the institutions that structure distributions of attention and resources, and inform social hierarchy.[4]

According to Raha and Van Der Drift, to be included in an institution, to be deemed worthy of its rights, is a double-edged sword. On the one hand, one gets access to certain resources controlled by the institution. However, on the other, one is now subject to the control of the institution. Think, for instance, of the position of the university lecturer. In being included by the institution (that is, employed by a university), the lecturer gains access to lots of resources controlled by the university: a wage, libraries, email lists, and so on. However, the lecturer is also now subject to the control of that institution: they must follow and even sometimes enforce its rules (no matter how morally troubling those rules are) or else lose their job.

Of course, existing outside of institutions right now (in what Raha and Van Der Drift call the realm of "chaos") doesn't exactly look very attractive either. Institutions like states and corporations control many of the resources that we need to live. So, Raha and Van Der Drift say let's abolish institutions! However, that doesn't mean that we all just exist as isolated individuals in the realm of chaos instead. Rather, Raha and Van Der Drift point to another way of organising social life that they see as preferable: the collective. Their model here is the shared transfemme forms of life that they have been a part of building in the UK and the Netherlands, respectively. These forms of life include practices of mutual aid and care, shared experiences, and aesthetics. Importantly, they also feature new forms of collective action, infrastructure, and production that would enable life outside and beyond the institution. So: we get access to the sorts of material and social resources that we need to live our lives without submitting to being controlled by institutions.

There's much to like about this sort of position. Given the violence and inequality faced by trans people, it's clear that *something* has to change to improve our lives, but what? Abolitionists like Raha and Van Der Drift give us a radical and urgent answer: virtually everything! The institutions that structure all of our lives need to be torn down, to be replaced by new social structures based around collectives.

However, it's not entirely clear that Raha and Van Der Drift have quite got everything right. I think that there they face at least three challenges: one from defenders of rights, one from the defenders of institutions, and one from those who (like Raha and Van Der Drift themselves) would like to see the end of institutions.

THE DEFENDER OF RIGHTS

The challenge from the defender of rights might run something like this: sure, it's true that some rights have been wrongly limited in scope, granted only to certain groups of people and only under certain conditions. That is, some states have implemented rights nonuniversally (say, through racialised slavery) or made rights conditional to following certain rules (say, through the implementation of the death penalty for certain crimes). However, such implementations of rights in policy were unjust or wrong. The slave has the moral right to be free, even if they live in a state that doesn't enforce that right through legal or political means.

This line of argument holds that, properly understood, moral rights are unconditional and universal. So, the right to not be killed or the right to freedom from slavery should be enjoyed by all without restriction. Here the thought is that one can do whatever one wants and still enjoy these fundamental moral rights. Even if one commits an egregious crime against humanity, one still has the right not to be enslaved or killed. Such moral rights do not involve submitting to forms of institutional control, we might think, and as such are defensible and worth fighting for.

Of course, one might respond here that an abstract moral right is useless without its implementation via a political mechanism (i.e., an institution guaranteeing that your right to be free from slavery is not violated) and hence requires at least *some* submission to institutional control. However, this sort of response to the defender of rights might not be available to Raha and Van Der Drift. They seem to see themselves as objecting to *both* the political rights that actually get enforced and the universal moral rights proposed by normative ethicists such Immanuel Kant, who is one of their main punching bags throughout their book. Moreover, why couldn't *collectives* be the ones to implement and guarantee rights?

THE DEFENDER OF INSTITUTIONS

The defender of institutions might make a few responses to Raha and Van Der Drift, but one is to suggest that Raha and Van Der Drift's objections to institutions apply only to certain institutions. Certainly, the defender of institutions might admit that many institutions are sites of control and violent boundary policing, not least in the literal boundary policing of modern state borders. However, there seem to be ways of organising institutions without such control and violence. Take, for instance, a public library that does not employ fines but rather stops a reader from borrowing further books until they have returned any late books that they have taken out. This seems like a non-violent institution, and while maybe this borrowing policy does count as a form of control, if it is a form of control, it is hardly an objectionable one. Institutions, then, are not the problem; instead, the problem is how some of them are organised and that some of them employ violence and objectionable forms of control.

THE OPPONENT OF INSTITUTIONS

Finally, those who Raha and Van Der Drift might normally think of as allies could also pose an objection. Those who agree that all institutions ought to be abolished might be a little suspicious of these things that Raha and Van Der Drift call 'collectives' and endorse as forms of social organisation that could replace institutions. What, after all, is the difference between institutions and collectives? Collectives are, for Raha and Van Der Drift, composed of individuals in direct relationships with one another and are often organised nonhierarchically, such that there are no formal leaders of collectives. The trouble is, of course, that the same thing can be said of many institutions! Whilst they are more likely to be organised hierarchically, there are some nonhierarchical institutions and even some hierarchical collectives.

So, what is the difference between a collective and an institution? One purported difference that Raha and Van Der Drift suggest is that leaving or refusing to participate in a collective indicates something different than leaving or refusing to participate in an institution. Why is this? Well, they think that in institutions are designed to function such that individual people who are a part of the can be replaced frictionlessly and their complaints ignored. Meanwhile, a good collective values those individuals more, and hence an individual leaving or ceasing to participate in the collective will create a great deal of friction, reflection, or disruption in the collective. Hence, they argue that someone leaving a collective indicates that things are not going well for the collective, whilst someone leaving an institution is taken as an indication that everything is going well for the institution.[5]

However, there are cases where this rule doesn't seem true. Think, for instance, of a massive strike at a factory due to poor management, with all of the workers putting down tools, refusing to participate, or even quitting their jobs. Here we have an institution (the factory) where refusal to participate or leaving the institution indicates massive managerial failure. Production will be massively disrupted, and however we slice it, things are not going well in the institution. Meanwhile, take a paradigmatic collective: a trans feminist art collective based in a town. Suppose one member of the collective is enjoying their art practice but needs to move across the country to look after a sick relative. That member thus leaves the collective without a fuss to attend to the relative. Now, this doesn't indicate that anything is going wrong in the art collective! So: institutions and collectives can both be affected by a person leaving them in both positive and negative ways, with varying degrees of friction on each.

Why does this matter? Well, if one is opposed to institutions, then unless one can find a principled way to distinguish between institutions and collectives, then it looks like one should also be opposed to collectives. So, Raha and Van Der Drift's commitment to collectives might be accused of 'betraying the revolution' by those who are opposed to institutions. Now, it may be that Raha and Van Der Drift can provide a way to set collectives apart from institutions. But perhaps the better approach is a more piecemeal one: rather than making general claims about institutions and collectives, we look at particular forms of social organisation and assess whether they are attractive or not. So, the question to ask is not whether institutions are in general objectionable but rather whether this particular squatting co-op, legal apparatus, or mode of production is objectionable and, if it is objectionable, to think about the particular ways to change it or the particular kind of social organisation we'd like to replace it if we think that it is irredeemable.

TRANSGENDER MARXISM

Even if we take a piecemeal approach to the evaluation of particular forms of social life, we can still keep the big picture in view. One way to approach thinking about institutions in this way is to think about the shifting role that particular institutions have played in broader society. Marxists, for instance, tend to focus on the role that such institutions play in economic production and class conflict. Take, for example, M.E. O'Brien. O'Brien, a trans Marxist, has developed an extensive history and critique of the family as one such institution. O'Brien describes the changing role and structure of the family under capitalism, arguing that overcoming the family is tied to overcoming capitalism. Instead of care being organised privately in the family, O'Brien argues for a communism that involves democratic and collective forms of care.[6]

Trans Marxists have been remarkably productive in the past decade or so, and there's not space here to recount the wide variety of ways that trans philosophers have drawn on Marx and Marxist thought to make sense of trans life under contemporary capitalism. It's perhaps worth drawing out some of the central themes in this tradition, however:

- A rejection of the idea that rights alone will liberate trans people. Whilst perhaps less openly *antagonistic* to rights than trans anarchists, trans Marxists tend to hold that such rights are insufficient without radical economic change.
- An emphasis on the economic and class situation of trans people. Noting the over-representation of trans women in sex work, for instance, trans Marxists have been keen to theorise how this economic position poses particular challenges and opportunities for political activity.
- A focus on the family as a part of economic production, its role in ensuring a steady supply of labour for capitalism, and as a fulcrum around which the marginalisation of trans people occurs.
- Like Prosser and Namaste, trans Marxists attempt to focus on "trans life as it is lived" rather than literary abstraction or ideal figures, with the aim of building political movements to achieve radical change.[7]

Of course, this broad set of commitments takes on a variety of different forms, and we've already seen some of their work in earlier chapters (e.g., Metcalfe on the why of transition).

Perhaps the most famous transgender Marxist was the author of *The Stone Butch Blues*, Leslie Feinberg. Feinberg's final words were "Remember me as a revolutionary communist"! Hir work is informed by a long tradition of working class and queer struggle and is particularly notable for the ways that sie draws on the history of trans resistance to capitalist exploitation. For instance, Feinberg points out that in the practice of enclosure in 17th-century England, resistance was led by an anonymous cross-dressing figure known as Lady Skimmington.[8] Enclosure was the process by which previously common land was privatised and taken away from the peasants as England transitioned from feudalism to capitalism. Riots erupted in response, with 'Lady Skimmingtons' appearing across south-west England at the head of the resistance. Amusingly, the state seems not to have realised that there was not one person called Lady Skimmington but rather many people taking on the role of Lady Skimmington. A search for 'the' Lady Skimmington was launched by a government that "feared that Skimmington was everywhere"![9] Meanwhile, Feinberg draws a direct line between 18th-century raids on London's queer 'Molly Clubs' and the New York Police's raids on contemporary queer bars like Stonewall:

> In London, some 300 years before the Stonewall Rebellion, police routinely raided "molly houses" – clubs frequented by feminine, cross-dressed males who were presumed to be gay. During one raid in London in 1725, the crowd – many of them in drag – fought pitched battles with the police.[10]

Why does Feinberg think that this sort of historical context is important? One answer might be this: that in pointing to the existence and resistance of trans people through time, trans people are able to make a rhetorical point: we have always been here, despite your attempts to repress us, and will always be here! This sort of thought can be quite personally empowering and serves as a counterpoint to the loneliness and isolation that can accompany being trans in an overwhelmingly cisgender world. However, this sort of move has its pitfalls: it can often lead to interminable debates over whether this or that historical figure was 'really' trans or 'would be trans if they were alive today'. Such debates, we might think, are irresolvable given that such figures are long dead.

Instead, Feinberg thinks that the history of this sort of resistance is important for a couple of other reasons. First, sie argues that we can look to the history of repression of gender nonconformity and diversity in order to understand where this sort of oppression comes from and how it relates to things like the rise of capitalism and colonialism. Second, sie suggests that looking at the history of resistance to that repression can teach us lessons for contemporary political activism.[11]

One of the crucial lessons for contemporary activism that Feinberg draws from this history is that trans people cannot do it alone: we need to build coalitions with other oppressed groups in order to fight for our liberation. In traditional Marxist thought, the oppressed class – known as the 'proletariat' – doesn't require any alliances with other groups. After all, the proletariat is the vast majority of people in society: it's the masses of people who work selling their labour to bosses for a wage. Meanwhile, trans people are a tiny minority, who do not have much leverage. As such, in many of hir speeches, Feinberg is keen to emphasise that trans people and other minorities need to work together as a coalition:

> "An injury to one is an injury to all". It's a truth the union movement was built on. It's a solid bedrock to build a lesbian, gay, bisexual, and transgender movement on, too. And it reminds us of our connection to others who are fighting for justice and equality.[12]

Feinberg lived out this idea in many ways, organising, writing, and marching for a variety of causes. For Feinberg, the struggle for Palestinian freedom, the fight against homophobia, and the end of police violence against Black Americans are all connected and are all worthy causes to stand in solidarity with. Whilst it's clear that sie thought that there was good moral reason for supporting each of these causes, Feinberg also thought that the history of liberation movements showed that failure to stand in solidarity with others led to their downfall.[13]

Exactly how to build what Feinberg was imagining – a coalition that brings together antiracist, working-class, decolonial, LGBTQ+, feminist, disability, and other movements besides – is still an open question. It seems clear, however, that it is not something that can be done solely from the philosopher's armchair. If trans political philosophers are to contribute anything to the practice of trans liberation in this radical tradition, it must be either learned from the history of such movements or as a part of the practice of activism and agitation, learning how to build coalitional movements through participation in them.

Trans political philosophy is a vast and growing subfield, one that we've only scratched the surface of here in this chapter. However, some general themes can be discerned: that trans political philosophy is radical in outlook and that trans political philosophers are keen to overthrow many, if not all of the institutions of contemporary society. As the repression of trans people around the world continues to ramp up, the trans political philosophy's calls for us to upend cisgender society look more and more urgent.

NOTES

1 Schuringa, Christoph. (2025). *A Social History of Analytic Philosophy*. London and New York: Verso.
2 Cousens, Emily. (2023). *Trans Feminist Epistemologies in the US Second Wave*. New York and London: Palgrave Macmillan.
3 Raha, Nat and Van Der Drift, Mijke. (2024). *Trans Femme Futures: Abolitionist Ethics for Transfeminist Worlds*. London: Pluto Press.
4 Raha and Van Der Drift, *Trans Femme Futures*, 81–82.
5 Raha and Van Der Drift, *Trans Femme Futures*, 83–84.
6 O'Brien, M.E. (2023). *Family Abolition: Capitalism and the Communizing of Care*. London: Pluto Press.
7 Gleeson, Jules Joanne and O'Rourke, Elle. (2021). "Introduction", in Jules Joanne Gleeson and Elle O'Rourke (eds.) *Transgender Marxism*. London: Pluto Press, p. 27.
8 Feinberg, Leslie. (1992). *Trans Gender Liberation: A Movement Whose Time Has Come*. New York: World View Forum, pp. 15–16.
9 Sharpe, Buchanan. (2010/1980). *In Contempt of All Authority: Rural Artisans and Riot in the West of England, 1586–1660*. London: Breviary Stuff, p. 68.
10 Feinberg, Leslie. (1998). *Transgender Liberation: Beyond Pink or Blue*. Boston: Beacon Press, p. 102.
11 Feinberg, *Transgender Liberation: Beyond Pink or Blue*, 123–124. See also Feinberg, *Trans Gender Liberation: A Movement Whose Time Has Come*.
12 Feinberg, *Transgender Liberation: Beyond Pink or Blue*, 103.
13 Feinberg, Leslie. (2002). "Speech at the Al-Fatiha Retreat". *coloursofresistance.org*. http://www.coloursofresistance.org/468/leslie-feinbergs-speech-at-the-al-fatiha-retreat/

RECOMMENDATIONS FOR FURTHER READING

One of the more powerful statements of a transfeminist political theory comes in Emi Koyama's 'Transfeminist Manifesto'. Koyama, like many of the thinkers surveyed here, is largely unconcerned with traditional topics in political philosophy and begins instead by thinking about the violence faced by trans women:

Koyama, Emi. (2003). "The Transfeminist Manifesto", in Rory Dicker and Alison Piepmeier (eds.) *Catching a Wave: Reclaiming Feminism for the 21st Century*. Boston: Northeastern University Press, pp. 244–259.

Whilst Marxist and anarchist perspectives are the rule in transgender political philosophy, there are some exceptions, especially in applied debates over things like gender markers on passports and sports policy. Heath Fogg Davis, for instance, explores applied policy issues through a (non-assimilationist) liberal anti-discrimination lens, whilst Rach Cosker-Rowland takes a rights-based approach:

Cosker-Rowland, Rach. (2025). "Freedom of Gender". *Journal of Ethics and Social Philosophy* 30(7): 1125–1170.

Davis, Heath Fogg. (2017). *Beyond Trans: Does Gender Matter.* New York: New York University Press.

Another thinker working in this broad tradition is Stephanie Kapusta:

Kapusta, Stephanie. (2019). "Transgender Rights", in Hugh LaFollette (ed.) *The International Encyclopedia of Ethics*. https://doi.org/10.1002/9781444367072.wbiee934

Kapusta, Stephanie. (2022). "Gender Autonomy", in Ben Colburn (ed.) *The Routledge Handbook of Autonomy*. London: Routledge, pp. 346–356.

Another place that more liberal political philosophy has been developed by transgender political philosophers is in their engagements with legal systems. A recent court case in the USA ruled that anti-employment discrimination policies protected LGBT people from discrimination. The ruling that the court offered mirrored the argument that had been submitted to the court by the philosophers Robin Dembroff and Issa Kohler-Hausmann:

Kohler-Hausmann, Issa. (2019). "Brief of the Philosophy Professors as Amici Curiae in Support of the Employees". Bostock v. Clayton County U.S. Supreme Court. https://www.supremecourt.gov/DocketPDF/17/17-1618/107015/20190703125853982_17-1618%2017-1623%2018-107%20PhilosophyProfessors%20Brief.pdf

In addition to rejecting centrist thought from the left, some trans people have taken up (rather esoteric) forms of right-wing political theory. For instance, right-wing forms of the radical philosophy known as accelerationism inspired the work of Nyx Land:

Land, Nyx. (2018). "Gender Acceleration: A Blackpaper". *Vastabrupt.com*. https://vastabrupt.com/2018/10/31/gender-acceleration/

GLOSSARY

Agender A lack of a gender identity, or a person with no gender.

Androgyne A non-binary gender that involves a blend of masculinity and femininity.

Bigender Someone who identifies as two genders, sometimes simultaneously, sometimes going back and forth.

Butch An identity emerging from American lesbian cultures that involves masculine presentation and gender expression.

Cis Abbreviated version of cisgender.

Cisgender A person whose gender identity matches the gender that they were assigned at birth.

Epistemology A subfield of philosophy concerned with issues to do with knowledge, including how we know things and the justification for our beliefs.

Ethics A subfield of philosophy concerned with what we should do and how we should live.

Fa'afāfine A Samoan gender, neither man nor woman, usually acknowledged in childhood by those assigned male at birth.

Gender-Affirming Treatment An array of hormonal, surgical, and other forms of medical care for trans people that allows them to access the sort of body that would make them feel most comfortable.

Gender Dysphoria The negative feelings such as distress, discomfort, unease, and so on that come from living in a body that does not match the gender identity that a person has. Similarly, the negative feelings that come from living in social roles and positions that do not match the gender identity that a person has. Additionally, a medical diagnosis of such feelings that has sometimes been used to determine who is transgender.

Gender Euphoria The positive feelings such as satisfaction, joy, 'feeling at home', comfort, and so on that come from living in a body that matches the gender identity that a person has. Similarly, the positive feelings that come from living social roles and positions that match the gender identity that a person has.

Gender Variant An extremely broad shorthand for anyone who lives in ways that deviate from dominant understandings of gender as binary and tied to sex.

Heterosexism A way of organising society that assumes that heterosexuality is the norm and that other forms of sexuality are deviant. Also: discrimination against non-heterosexual people based on the idea that heterosexuality is normal or preferable in comparison to other sexualities.

Hijra A South Asian gender, with a wide variety of social roles and understandings across the subcontinent.

Ideology A widespread set of related beliefs and practices. Usually used to refer pejoratively to a society's dominant and morally troubling ways of thinking about and organising some part of social life.

If and only if A 'biconditional' composed of two 'if. . . then . . .' statements placed back to back, e.g., 'X is a duck if and only if X quacks' is true only when 'if X is a duck, then it quacks' is true and 'if X quacks, then it is a duck' is true. Sometimes written as 'iff'.

Intersex Intersex people are those people who are born with bodies that don't fit a binary understanding of sex. This might involve them having a chromosomal makeup other than XX or XY or involve genitalia that don't look like the 'usual' male and female types.

Kind A grouping of things in the world, e.g., *tiger*, *iPod*, and *woman*. Kinds have members: the kind *tiger*'s members are all of the actual tigers out there in the world.

Metaphysics A subfield of philosophy concerned with questions about existence, including what exists, how things exist, and how those things are related to one another.

Misgendering The treatment of a person as not having the gender with which they identify.

Nonbinary A gender that is neither man nor woman. Sometimes used as an umbrella category to include identities like *androgyne*, *bigender*, and *genderfluid*, sometimes used as a distinct gender identity of its own.

Patriarchy A social structure, or way of organising society, that privileges men over women and ensures men's continued dominance in that society.

Phenomenology As used in this book, what it is like to experience something or what it is like to be something. Additionally, a subfield of philosophy that emerged in the early 20th century, largely concerned with studying the basic structures of experience.

Trans Abbreviated version of *transgender*.

Transfemme/Transfeminine A trans person who expresses their gender in a feminine way or whose gender is in some way feminine.

Transgender Usually, a person whose gender identity does not match the gender that they were assigned at birth. Occasionally used to refer to a broader category of gender variant people.

Transmasc/Transmasculine A trans person who expresses their gender in a masculine way or whose gender is in some way masculine.

Transmisogyny Discrimination against, prejudice towards, and oppression of trans women.

Transsexual An identity adopted by many trans people who have undertaken hormonal and/or surgical interventions to change their body to better align with their gender identity.

Trans man Someone who identifies as a man but who was not assigned male at birth.

Trans woman Someone who identifies as a woman but who was not assigned female at birth.

BIBLIOGRAPHY

Alcoff, Linda Martin. (1988). "Cultural Feminism Versus Post-Structuralism: The Identity Crisis in Feminist Theory". *Signs* 13(3): 408.

Ashley, Florence. (2021). "Accounting for Research Fatigue in Research Ethics". *Bioethics* 35: 270–276.

Ashley, Florence. (2023). "What is it Like to Have a Gender Identity?". *Mind* 132(528): 1053–1073.

Ásta. (2018). *Categories We Live By: The Construction of Race, Gender, and Other Social Categories*. Oxford: Oxford University Press.

Awkward-Rich, Cameron. (2022). *The Terrible We: Thinking with Trans Maladjustment*. Durham: Duke University Press.

Bailey, Moya. (2021). *Misogynoir Transformed: Black Women's Digital Resistance*. United States: NYU Press.

Baldwin, James. (1998). "Freaks and the American Ideal of Manhood", in Toni Morrison (ed.) *James Baldwin: Collected Essays*. New York: Library of America, pp. 814–829.

Barnes, Elizabeth. (2019). "Gender and Gender Terms". *Noûs* 54(3): 704–730.

Barnes, Elizabeth. (2022). "Gender Without Gender Identity: The Case of Cognitive Disability". *Mind* 131(523): 836–862.

Barthes, Roland. (1977). "The Death of the Author", in Stephen Heath (trans.) *Image Music Text*. London: HarperCollins, pp. 142–148.

Beauvoir, Simone de. (1949/2011). *The Second Sex*, Constance Borde and Sheila Malovany-Chevallier (trans.). London: Vintage Books.

Belinsky, Zoe. (2019). "Gender and Family Abolition as an Expansive and Not Reductive Process". *medium.com*. https://medium.com/@

malkekvmachashayfele/gender-and-family-abolition-as-an-expansive-and-not-reductive-process-d933f1f71da2 (accessed 24 October 2022).

Benjamin, Harry. (1966/1999). *The Transsexual Phenomenon*. Düsseldorf: Symposium.

Berkins, Lohana. (2019). *Selected Writings*, Jamie Berrout (trans.). River Furnace. https://www.patreon.com/posts/full-text-of-26491264

Berson, Ginny. (2020). *Olivia on the Record: A Radical Experiment in Women's Music*. California: Aunt Lute Books.

Bettcher, Talia Mae. (2019). "What is Trans Philosophy?". *Hypatia* 34(4): 644–667.

Bettcher, Talia Mae. (2007). "Evil Deceivers and Make Believers: On Transphobic Violence and the Politics of Illusion". *Hypatia* 22(3): 43–65.

Bettcher, Talia Mae. (2009). "Trans Identities and First-Person Authority", in Laurie Schrage (ed.) *You've Changed: Sex Reassignment and Personal Identity*. Oxford: Oxford University Press, pp. 98–120.

Bettcher, Talia Mae. (2013). "Trans Women and the Meaning of 'Woman'", in A. Soble, N. Power and R. Halwani (eds.) *Philosophy of Sex: Contemporary Readings*, 6th edn. Plymouth: Rowan and Littlefield, pp. 233–250.

Bettcher, Talia Mae. (2014). "Trapped in the Wrong Theory: Rethinking Trans Oppression and Resistance". *Signs: Journal of Women in Culture and Society* 39(2): 383–406.

Bettcher, Talia Mae. (2025). *Beyond Personhood: An Essay in Trans Philosophy*. Minneapolis: University of Minnesota Press.

Binaohan, B. (2014). *Decolonizing Trans/Gender 101*. Toronto: Biyuti Publishing.

Bjegunac, Stani. (2019). "Trans-cending the Market: How Socialist Planning Can Meet the Needs of Transgender People". *Cosmonaut Magazine*. https://cosmonautmag.com/2019/09/trans-cending-the-market-how-socialist-planning-can-meet-the-needs-of-transgender-people/ (accessed 24 October 2022).

Blanchard, R. (1989). "The Concept of Autogynephilia and the Typology of Male Gender Dysphoria". *The Journal of Nervous and Mental Disease* 177(10): 616–623.

Briggs, R.A. (2023). "Normative Theories of Rational Choice: Expected Utility". *Stanford Encyclopedia of Philosophy*. https://plato.stanford.edu/entries/rationality-normative-utility/

Briggs, R.A. and George, B.R. (2023). *What Even is Gender?*. Abingdon and New York: Routledge.

Burman, Åsa. (2023). *Nonideal Social Ontology: The Power View*. New York: Oxford University Press.

Butler, Judith. (1999). *Gender Trouble: Tenth Anniversary Edition*. Routledge.

Butler, Judith. (2004). *Undoing Gender*. Abingdon: Routledge.

Campuzano, Giuseppe. (2006). "Reclaiming Travesti Histories". *IDS Bulletin* 37(5): 34–39.

cárdenas, micha. (2016). "Pregnancy: Reproductive Futures in Trans of Color Feminism". *TSQ* 3(1–2): 48–57.

Chan, Rebecca. (2023). "Transformative Experience". *Stanford Encyclopedia of Philosophy*. https://plato.stanford.edu/entries/transformative-experience

Chappell, Sophie-Grace. (2025). *Trans Figured: On Being a Transgender Person in a Cisgender World*. Bristol: Polity.

Chu, Andrea Long. (2019). *Females*. London and New York: Verso.

Chu, Andrea Long and Harsin Drager, Emmett. (2019). "After Trans Studies". *TSQ* 6(1): 103–116.

Corvino, John. (2000). "Analyzing Gender". *Southwest Philosophy Review* 17(1): 173–180.

Cosker-Rowland, Rach. (2023). "Recent Work on Gender Identity and Gender". *Analysis* 83 (4): 801–820.

Cosker-Rowland, Rach. (2025). "Freedom of Gender". *Journal of Ethics and Social Philosophy* 30(7): 1125–1170.

Cosker-Rowland, Rach. (2025). *Gender Identity: What it is and Why it Matters*. Oxford: Oxford University Press.

Cousens, Emily. (2023). *Trans Feminist Epistemologies in the US Second Wave*. New York and London: Palgrave Macmillan.

Crenshaw, Kimberlé. (2017). *On Intersectionality: Essential Writings*. New York: The New Press.

Cull, Matthew J. (Forthcoming). "Children as Commodity and Changeling: Gender Disappointments and Gender Disappointment!", in Matthew Cull, Alexis Davin and Katharine Jenkins (eds.) *Trans Philosophy in a Time of Crisis*. London and New York: Bloomsbury.

Cull, Matthew J. (2019). "Against Abolition". *Feminist Philosophy Quarterly* 5(3).

Cull, Matthew J. (2022). "Epistemic Injustice and Trans Lives", in Laura Erikson-Scroth (ed.) *Trans Bodies, Trans Selves*, 2nd edn. Oxford: Oxford University Press, pp. 656–657.

Cull, Matthew J. (2024a). "Queer Identities in Political Contexts", in Julie A. Gedro and Tonette S. Rocco (eds.) *The Routledge Companion to LGBTQ Identity in Global, Social, Political, and Work Contexts*. Abingdon: Routledge, pp. 365–376.

Cull, Matthew J. (2024b). "Un Œuf but Enough: Trans Epistemology and Methodological Radicalism". *Hypatia* 39(1): 44–60.

Cull, Matthew J. (2024c). *What Gender Should Be*. London: Bloomsbury.

Cull, Matthew J. (2025). "Ideal Theory, Literary Theory, Whither Transfeminism?", in Hilkje Charlotte Hänel and Johanna M. Müller (eds.) *The Routledge Handbook of Non-Ideal Theory*. New York: Routledge, pp. 246–258.

Cull, Matthew J. (2026). "A Plea for Pluralism". *Transgender Studies Quarterly* 13(2): 222–227.

Cull, Matthew J., Holroyd, Jules and Woollard, Fiona. (2025). "Caring for Everyone: Effective and Inclusive Communication in Perinatal Care". *Hypatia* 40(3): 525–546.

Davis, Heath Fogg. (2017). *Beyond Trans: Does Gender Matter.* New York: New York University Press.

Dembroff, Robin. (2018). "Real Talk on the Metaphysics of Gender". *Philosophical Topics* 46(2): 21–50.

Dembroff, Robin. (2020). "Beyond Binary: Genderqueer as Critical Gender Kind". *Philosopher's Imprint* 20(9): 1–23.

DeVun, Leah. (2021). *The Shape of Sex: Nonbinary Gender from Genesis to the Renaissance.* New York: Columbia University Press.

Díaz-León, Esa. (2016). "Woman as a Politically Significant Term: A Solution to the Puzzle". *Hypatia* 31(2): 245–258.

DiPietro, P.J. (2025). *Sideways Selves: Travesti and Jotería Struggles Across the Américas.* Texas: University of Texas Press.

Djelid, Aisha. (2024). "'The Master Whished to Reproduce': Slavery, Forced Intimacy, and Enslavers' Interference in Sexual Relationships in the Antebellum South, 1808–1861". *American Nineteenth Century History* 25(1): 21–43.

Du Bois, W.E.B. (1897/1970). "The Conservation of Races", in Philip S. Foner (ed.) *W. E. B. Du Bois Speaks: Speeches and Addresses, 1890–1919.* New York: Pathfinder Press.

Ellison, Treva, Green, Kai M., Richardson, Matt and Snorton, C. Riley (eds.). (2017). "The Issue of Blackness". *Transgender Studies Quarterly* 4(2).

Escalante, Alyson. (2016). "Gender Nihilism: An Anti-Manifesto". *libcom.org.* https://libcom.org/article/gender-nihilism-anti-manifesto-alyson-escalante

Feinberg, Leslie. (1992). *Trans Gender Liberation: A Movement Whose Time Has Come.* New York: World View Forum.

Feinberg, Leslie. (1998). *Transgender Liberation: Beyond Pink or Blue.* Boston: Beacon Press.

Feinberg, Leslie. (2002). "Speech at the Al-Fatiha Retreat". *coloursofresistance.org.* http://www.coloursofresistance.org/468/leslie-feinbergs-speech-at-the-al-fatiha-retreat/

Firestone, Shulamith. (1970). *The Dialectic of Sex: The Case for Feminist Revolution.* New York: William Morrow.

Flint, C., Förster, K., Koser, S.A. et al. 2020. "Biological Sex Classification with Structural MRI Data Shows Increased Misclassification in Transgender Women". *Neuropsychopharmacology* 45: 1758–1765.

Freud, Sigmund. (1953). *The Standard Edition of the Complete Psychological Works of Sigmund Freud Volume VII*, James Strachey, Anna Freud, Alix Strachey and Alan Tyson (trans.). London: The Hogarth Press.

Fricker, Miranda. (2007). *Epistemic Injustice: Power and the Ethics of Knowing*. Oxford: Oxford University Press.

Fricker, Miranda and Jenkins, Katharine. (2017). "Epistemic Injustice, Ignorance, and Trans Experiences", in Ann Garry, Serene J. Khader and Alison Stone (eds.) *The Routledge Companion to Feminist Philosophy*. New York and London: Routledge, pp. 268–278.

George, B.R. and Briggs, R.A. (unpublished). "Science Fiction Double Feature: Trans Liberation on Twin Earth". https://philpapers.org/archive/GEOSFD.pdf

George, B.R. and Stacey, Goguen. (2021). "Hermeneutical Backlash: Trans Youth Panics as Epistemic Injustice". *Feminist Philosophy Quarterly* 7(4).

Gertler, Brie. (2021). "Self-Knowledge", in Edward N. Zalta (ed.) *The Stanford Encyclopedia of Philosophy (Winter 2021 Edition)*. https://plato.stanford.edu/archives/win2021/entries/self-knowledge/

Gleeson, Jules Joanne. (2021). "How Do Gender Transitions Happen?", in Jules Joanne Gleeson and Elle O'Rourke (eds.) *Transgender Marxism*. London: Pluto Press, pp. 70–84.

Gleeson, Jules Joanne and O'Rourke, Elle. (2021). "Introduction", in Jules Joanne Gleeson and Elle O'Rourke (eds.) *Transgender Marxism*. London: Pluto Press, pp. 1–32.

Gleeson, Juliana. (2025). *Hermaphrodite Logic: A History of Intersex Liberation*. London and New York: Verso.

Goetze, Trystan S. (2018). "Hermeneutical Dissent and the Species of Hermeneutical Injustice". *Hypatia* 33(1): 73–90.

Gregory, Andrew. (2025). "'Concerning' Lack of Female-Only Medical Trials in UK, Say Health Experts". *theguardian.com*. https://www.theguardian.com/society/2025/may/07/concerning-lack-of-female-only-medical-trials-in-uk-say-health-experts (accessed 23 December 2025).

Halberstam, Jack. (1994). "F2M: The Making of Female Masculinity", in L. Doan (ed.) *The Lesbian Postmodern*. New York: Columbia University Press, pp. 210–228.

Hale, C. Jacob. (1996). "Are Lesbians Women?". *Hypatia* 11(2): 94–120.

Haslanger, Sally. (2000). "Gender and Race: (What) are They? (What) Do We Want Them to Be?". *Noûs* 34(1): 31–55.

Henckel, S.J. (2025). "You Think You Know Someone: Trans Identities and Epistemic Injustice". *Hypatia*, first look: 1–22.

Hernandez, E.M. (Forthcoming). "Fuel to My Fire/You Can't Stop Desire", in Matthew Cull, Alexis Davin and Katharine Jenkins (eds.) *Trans Philosophy in a Time of Crisis*. London and New York: Bloomsbury.

Hernandez, E.M. (2024). "Moral Shock and Trans 'Worlds' of Sense". *Journal of the American Philosophical Association* 10(4): 761–779.

Hernandez, E.M. and Bell, Rowan. (2025). "Much Ado About Nothing: Unmotivating 'Gender Identity'". *Ergo: An Open Access Journal of Philosophy* 12(50): 1313–1340.

Hester, Helen. (2018). *Xenofeminism*. Polity Press.

Heyes, Cressida. (2000). *Line Drawings: Defining Woman Through Feminist Practice*. Ithaca and New York: Cornell University Press.

Hume, David. (1739/1896). *A Treatise of Human Nature*. Oxford: Clarendon Press.

Ivy, Veronica (authored as Rachel McKinnon). (2015). "Trans*Formative Experiences". *Res Philosophica* 92(2): 219–440.

Jaggar, Alison. (1983). *Feminist Politics and Human Nature*. Sussex: Harvester Press.

James, L. (ed.). (1997). *Women, Men, and Eunuchs: Gender in Byzantium*. Abingdon: Routledge.

Jenkins, Katharine. (2016). "Amelioration and Inclusion: Gender Identity and the Concept of Woman". *Ethics* 126(2): 403–404.

Jenkins, Katharine. (2018). "Toward an Account of Gender Identity". *Ergo* 5(27). https://doi.org/10.3998/ergo.12405314.0005.027

Jenkins, Katharine. (2023). *Ontology and Oppression: Race, Gender, and Social Reality*. Oxford: Oxford University Press.

Jesperson, Jamey. (2024). "Trans Misogyny in the Colonial Archive: Re-membering Trans Feminine Life and Death in New Spain, 1604–1821". *Gender & History* 36: 91–111.

Kapusta, Stephanie. (2019). "Transgender Rights", in Hugh LaFollette (ed.) *The International Encyclopedia of Ethics*. https://doi.org/10.1002/9781444367072.wbiee934

Kapusta, Stephanie. (2022). "Gender Autonomy", in Ben Colburn (ed.) *The Routledge Handbook of Autonomy*. London: Routledge, pp. 346–356.

Kapusta, Stephanie Julia. (2016). "Misgendering and Its Moral Contestability". *Hypatia* 31(3): 502–519.

Kierkegaard, Søren. (2009). *Concluding Unscientific Manuscript*. Cambridge: Cambridge University Press.

Killmister, Suzi. (2025). "What's Wrong with Gender-Critical Feminism?". *Hypatia*, first look: 1–22.

Kingma, Elselijn. (2019). "Were You a Part of Your Mother?". *Mind* 128(511): 609–646.

Kohler, Hausmann. (2019). "Brief of the Philosophy Professors as Amici Curiae in Support of the Employees". Bostock v. Clayton County U.S. Supreme Court. https://www.supremecourt.gov/DocketPDF/17/17-1618/107015/20190703125853982_17-1618%2017-1623%2018-107%20Philosophy Professors%20Brief.pdf

Koyama, Emi. (2003). "The Transfeminist Manifesto", in Rory Dicker and Alison Piepmeier (eds.) *Catching a Wave: Reclaiming Feminism for the 21st Century*. Boston: Northeastern University Press, pp. 244–259.

Kukla, Quill and Lance, Mark. (2022). "Telling Gender: The Pragmatics and Ethics of Gender Ascriptions". *Ergo* 9(42): 1130–1131.

Land, Nyx. (2018). "Gender Acceleration: A Blackpaper". *Vastabrupt.com*. https://vastabrupt.com/2018/10/31/gender-acceleration/

Le Guin, Ursula K. (2000). *The Left Hand of Darkness*. New York: Ace Books.

Lugones, María. (2010). "Toward a Decolonial Feminism". *Hypatia* 25(4): 742–759.

Mackinnon, Catharine A. (1989). *Toward a Feminist Theory of the State*. Cambridge, MA: Harvard University Press.

Male, Andrew. (2020). "'Our Sound Engineer got a Death Threat': How Lesbian Label Olivia Shook up Music". *The Guardian*. https://www.theguardian.com/music/2020/jul/19/lesbian-record-label-olivia-linda-tillery-californian-feminists-death-threat-music

McGlynn, Aidan. (2026). *Epistemic Injustice: An Introduction*. New York and London: Routledge.

McKitrick, Jennifer. (2015). "A Dispositional Account of Gender". *Philosophical Studies* 172(10): 2575–2589.

McLemore, K.A. (2018). "A Minority Stress Perspective on Transgender Individuals' Experiences with Misgendering". *Stigma and Health* 3(1): 53–64. https://doi.org/10.1037/sah0000070

Metcalfe, Xandra. (2021). "'Why are We Like This?' The Primacy of Transsexuality", in Jules Joanne Gleeson and Elle O'Rourke (eds.) *Transgender Marxism*. London: Pluto Press, pp. 219–229.

Mieli, Mario. (2018). *Towards a Gay Communism: Elements of a Homosexual Critique*, David Fernbach and Evan Calder Williams (trans.). London: Pluto Press.

Mikkola, Mari. (2016). *The Wrong of Injustice: Dehumanization and Its Role in Feminist Philosophy*. Oxford: Oxford University Press.

Mitchell, John Cameron. (2001). *Hedwig and the Angry Inch*. New Line Cinema. (Film)

More, Kate and Whittle, Stephen (eds.). (1999). *Reclaiming Genders: Transsexual Grammars at the Fin de Siècle*. London and New York: Cassell.

Morgensen, Scott Lauria. (2011). *Spaces Between Us*. Minneapolis: University of Minnesota Press.

Nagel, Thomas. (1979). "What it is Like to Be a Bat?". *Philosophical Review* 83(4): 430–450.

Namaste, Viviane. (2000). *Invisible Lives: The Erasure of Transsexual and Transgendered People*. Chicago and London: University of Chicago Press

NHS. (2022). "Gender Identity", in *Data Quality of Protected Characteristics and Other Vulnerable Groups*. https://digital.nhs.uk/data-and-information/data-collections-and-data-sets/data-sets/mental-health-services-data-set/submit-data/data-quality-of-protected-characteristics-and-other-vulnerable-groups/gender-identity (accessed 09 January 2024).

Nicholas, Harry. (2023). *A Trans Man Walks into a Gay Bar: A Journey of Self (and Sexual) Discovery*. London and Philadelphia: Jessica Kingsley.

O'Brien, M.E. (2023). *Family Abolition: Capitalism and the Communizing of Care*. London: Pluto Press.

Overall, Christine. (2009). "Sex/Gender Transitions and Life-Changing Aspirations", in Laurie Shrage (ed.) *You've Changed: Sex Reassignment and Personal Identity*. Oxford: Oxford University Press, pp. 11–27.

Paul, L.A. (2014). *Transformative Experience*. Oxford: Oxford University Press.

Pearce, Ruth. (2018). *Understanding Trans Health: Discourse, Power and Possibility*. Bristol: Polity.

Plato. (1989). *Symposium*, Alexander Nehamas and Paul Woodruff (trans.). Indianapolis and Cambridge: Hackett.

Pratt, Richard Henry. (1892). "The Advantages of Mingling Indians with Whites", in Isabel C. Barrows (ed.) *The Proceedings of the National Conference of Charities and Correction*. Geo H. Ellis: Boston, pp. 45–59.

Preciado, Paul B. (2000/2018). *Countersexual Manifesto*, Kevin Gerry Dunn (trans.). New York: Columbia University Press.

Preciado, Paul B. (2013). *Testo Junkie: Sex, Drugs, and Biopolitics in the Pharmacopornographic Era*. New York: Feminist Press.

Preciado, Paul B. (2021). *Can the Monster Speak?*, Frank Wynne (trans.). London: Fitzcarraldo.

Prosser, Jay. (1998). *Second Skins: The Body Narratives of Transsexuality*. New York: Columbia University Press.

Radi, Blas, Vlaad, Sofie, Wong, Jules and Bell, Rowan. (2026). "On Trans Philosophy's Methods: A Roundtable". *Transgender Studies Quarterly* 13(2): 228–245.

Raha, Nat and Van Der Drift, Mijke. (2024). *Trans Femme Futures: Abolitionist Ethics for Transfeminist Worlds*. London: Pluto Press.

Raymond, Janice. (1994). *The Transsexual Empire: The Making of the She-Male*. New York and London: Teachers Press.

Rea, Michael. (2022). "Gender as Self-Conferred Identity". *Feminist Philosophy Quarterly* 8(2).

Richardson, Kevin. (2022). "Exclusion and Erasure: Two Types of Ontological Oppression". *Ergo* 9(23): 603–622.

Rothblatt, Martine A. (1995). *The Apartheid of Sex: A Manifesto on the Freedom of Gender*. New York: Crown Publishing.

Salah, Trish. (2017). "What Does Tiresias Want?". *Transgender Studies Quarterly* 4(3–4): 632–638.

Saul, Jennifer. (2012). "Politically Significant Terms and Philosophy of Language: Methodological Issues", in Sharon Crasnow and Anita Superson (eds.) *Out from the Shadows: Analytical Feminist Contributions to Traditional Philosophy*. Oxford: Oxford University Press.

Schuringa, Christoph. (2025). *A Social History of Analytic Philosophy*. London and New York: Verso.

Serano, Julia. (2010). "The Case Against Autogynephilia". *International Journal of Transgenderism* 12(3): 176–187.

Serano, Julia. (2016). *Whipping Girl: A Transsexual Woman on Sexism and the Scapegoating of Femininity*, 2nd edn. Berkeley: Seal Press.

Sharpe, Buchanan. (2010/1980). *In Contempt of All Authority: Rural Artisans and Riot in the West of England, 1586–1660*. London: Breviary Stuff.

Silver, Kenneth. (2026). "The Standing of Self-Identity". *Hypatia* First View: 1–22.

Silver, Kenneth. (2018). "Do I Think Corporations Should Be Able to Vote Now?". *Journal of Business Ethics Review* 6(4): 18–23.

Simonetto, Patricio and Salvador, Vidal-Ortiz. (2025). "Lohana Berkins: A Latin American *Travesti* Theory of the Body". *Body and* Society 31(3): 3–27.

Snorton, C. Riley. (2017). *Black on Both Sides: A Racial History of Trans Identity*. Minneapolis: University of Minnesota Press.

Spillers, Hortense. (1987). "Mama's Baby, Papa's Maybe: An American Grammar Book". *Diacritics* 17(2): 65–81.

Stone, Sandy. (1993). "The Empire Strikes Back: A Posttranssexual Manifesto". *sandystone.com*. https://sandystone.com/empire-strikes-back.pdf

Stryker, Susan. (1994). "My Words to Victor Frankenstein Above the Village of Chamounix: Performing Transgender Rage". *GLQ* 1(3): 237–254.

Talusan, Meredith, Tobia, Jacob, Milan, Tiq and Nico, Fonseca. (2016). "Telling Trans Stories Beyond 'Born in the Wrong Body'". *Buzzfeed.com*. https://www.buzzfeed.com/meredithtalusan/telling-trans-stories-beyond-born-in-the-wrong-body

Truth and Reconciliation Commission of Canada. (2015). "Honouring the Truth, Reconciling for the Future Summary of the Final Report of the Truth and Reconciliation Commission of Canada". Publications of the Government of Canada. https://publications.gc.ca/collections/collection_2015/trc/IR4-7-2015-eng.pdf (accessed 19 December 2025).

Upadhyay, Nishant. (2021). "Coloniality of White Feminism and Its Transphobia: A Comment on Burt". *Feminist Criminology* 16(4): 539–544.

Weltman, Daniel. (2024). "What Do We Want? To Eliminate Gender! When Do We Want it? Later!". *Pacific Philosophical Quarterly* 105: 510–540.

Wilchins, Riki. (1997). *Read My Lips: Sexual Subversion and the End of Gender.* New York: Magnus Books.

Wynter, Sylvia. (2003). "Unsettling the Coloniality of Being/Power/Truth/ Freedom: Towards the Human, After Man, Its Overrepresentation – An Argument". *CR: The New Centennial Review* 3(3): 257–337.

Zapatista Women. (2019). "Letter from Zapatistas to Women Who Fight All Over the World", Abolition Media Worldwide (trans.). *InternationalViewpoint.org.* https://internationalviewpoint.org/spip.php?article5944 (accessed 19 December 2025).

Zurn, Perry. (2024). "Trans Philosophy", in *Stanford Encyclopedia of Philosophy.* https://plato.stanford.edu/entries/trans/ (accessed 18 December 2025).

INDEX

www.ingramcontent.com/pod-product-compliance
Lightning Source LLC
LaVergne TN
LVHW021300151026
850117LV00030B/306
9781032806570